Contents

Stroke

Your Complete Exercise Guide

The Cooper Clinic and Research Institute Fitness Series

Neil F. Gordon, MD, PhD, MPH
The Cooper Institute for Aerobics Research
Dallas, Texas

To Mom, Dad, Jenny, Jonny, Alan, and Rosie—with love

Library of Congress Cataloging-in-Publication Data

Gordon, Neil F.
    Stroke: your complete exercise guide / Neil F. Gordon.
        p.   cm.
    Includes index.
    ISBN 0-87322-428-0
    1. Cerebrovascular disease--Exercise therapy.   I. Title
  RC388.5.G67   1993
  616.8'1--dc20   92-39742
                                              CIP

ISBN: 0-87322-428-0

Human Kinetics books are available at special discounts for bulk purchase. Special editions or book exceprts can also be created to specification. For details, contact the Special Sales Manager at Human Kinetics.

Printed in the United States of America

10 9 8 7 6 5 4 3 2 1

Human Kinetics Publishers
Box 5076, Champaign, IL 61825-5076
1-800-747-4457

Canada: Human Kinetics Publishers, P.O. Box 2503, Windsor, ON N8Y 4S2
1-800-465-7301 (in Canada only)

Europe: Human Kinetics Publishers (Europe) Ltd., P.O. Box IW14,
Leeds LS16 6TR, England
0532-781708

Australia: Human Kinetics Publishers, P.O. Box 80, Kingswood 5062,
South Australia
618-374-0433

New Zealand: Human Kinetics Publishers, P.O. Box 105-231, Auckland 1
(09) 309-2259

Foreword

Each book in The Cooper Clinic and Research Institute Fitness Series covers an exercise rehabilitation program we devised to help our patients and other patients around the world recover from a chronic disorder. The series covers diabetes, chronic fatigue, breathing disorders, arthritis, and stroke.

I anticipate that the stroke patients who read this book will be highly motivated fighters—people who aren't going to let their situations, frustrating though they may sometimes be, get the best of them. They're going to do what needs to be done to keep on persevering with life—and with exercise. If you've got perseverance and you're determined to feel better, you've got the right book in your hands. My staff at The Cooper Aerobics Center* and I have developed what I believe is one of America's finest and safest exercise rehabilitation programs for stroke patients.

---

*The Cooper Aerobics Center, founded by Ken Cooper in Dallas in the early 1970s, is composed of the Cooper Clinic, a preventive and rehabilitative medicine facility; The Cooper Institute for Aerobics Research, where researchers study the role of exercise and other lifestyle factors in the maintenance of health; the Cooper Wellness Program, which provides a supportive, live-in environment where participants can focus time and attention on the challenging task of how to make positive lifestyle changes; and the Cooper Fitness Center, a health club in which all members' exercise efforts are supervised by a well-trained staff of health professionals.

Here you'll find a game plan for easing yourself into a regular exercise regimen. This book takes up where your formal 3-to 6-month stroke treatment and rehabilitation program leaves off. It is at this critical time when physical, speech, and occupational therapies terminate that an exercise program should begin, not end. Unfortunately, stroke survivors often receive little direction at this vital time in their rehabilitation, and that's one reason this book was written.

Our purpose in formulating the exercise program described in this book was twofold: to help restore patients to full functional capacity so they can live the rest of their lives as productive members of society and, equally important, to help them prevent another stroke as well as such chronic ailments as heart disease. There is one caveat, however. This book was written for people whose formal stroke rehabilitation program has brought them to the stage where only a slight to moderate disability remains, or none at all. This is not to say that those of you with a more severe disability won't benefit from what we have to say here. It's just that you'll need more detailed guidance and supervision from your doctor and other members of your health-care team in implementing an exercise program.

Stroke doesn't make the headlines as heart disease, cancer, or AIDS does, but it's a serious, ever-present health problem nonetheless. The statistics for the United States[1, 2] are startling: Stroke is the third leading cause of death, after heart disease and all types of cancer combined. In 1989, the most recent year for which the American Heart Association has provided figures, strokes killed 147,470 people. Each year, about half a million people will have a stroke, and about a quarter of them will be middle-aged people between 45 and 65 years old. Sixty-two percent of those who have strokes survive and join the almost 3 million people today whose medical records show that they've had one or more strokes.

The good news is that stroke death rates are shrinking in the United States and in most other industrialized nations, with the sad exception of Eastern European countries. Each year between 1970 and 1985, stroke death rates in the United States decreased, on average, by more than 5%.[3] Epidemiologists attribute this decline to three factors: Today, people with high blood pressure, an important risk factor for stroke, are more likely to have this condition under control. Similarly, people are more health-conscious and concerned about preventive medicine; they are informed about the lifestyle risk factors that stroke and heart disease share and are trying to exercise more and eat better. Finally, medical treatment for stroke patients has improved markedly.

However, it's because the need for a continuing, lifelong exercise program is not emphasized enough in the available books on stroke that we felt it necessary to write this one. What this book offers that others don't is comprehensive, state-of-the-art advice for patients who are largely recovered from a stroke on how to persevere and succeed in an exercise program. It tells you how to figure out just how much exercise is enough to improve health without increasing the risk of injury or other health problems.

I believe people need all the motivation they can get to break a bad health habit and replace it with a good one. To give you a strong incentive to maintain your health through regular exertion (while avoiding the aspects of exercise that are risky for stroke patients), this book comes complete with a Health Points System. It's a great system designed to keep you exercising over the long haul. It will ease you into a healthier lifestyle and motivate you to keep going, even on those days when you feel most tempted to backslide.

It's my hope that this book will serve as a springboard for discussions about exercise between you and your doctor. I also hope it will make you more self-sufficient and less dependent on your physician for all the small details of how to work exercise into your daily routine. But, I don't want you to ever regard our advice as a substitute for that of your doctor or any other health-care practitioner familiar with your case.

Stroke management has come a long way over the years. Today, most stroke patients can be rehabilitated. Given the tools—one of which is regular exercise—they can exert more control over their condition than ever before. As you read this book, you may discover you can partially—or almost fully—reverse some of the disabilities your stroke has triggered and, thus, return to a more active lifestyle. Cheer up. You may have far more control over your condition than you ever thought possible!

Kenneth H. Cooper, MD, MPH

About the Author

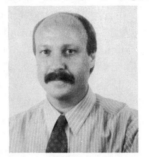

Dr. Neil F. Gordon is widely regarded as a leading medical authority on exercise and health. Before receiving his master's degree in public health from the University of California at Los Angeles in 1989, Dr. Gordon received doctoral degrees in exercise physiology and medicine at the University of the Witwatersrand in Johannesburg, South Africa. He also served as medical director of cardiac rehabilitation and exercise physiology for 6 years at I Military Hospital in Pretoria, South Africa.

Since 1987, Dr. Gordon has been the director of exercise physiology at the internationally renowned Cooper Institute for Aerobics Research in Dallas, Texas. He has also written over 50 papers related to exercise and medicine. Dr. Gordon is also coauthor of the book *Don't Count Yourself Out: Staying Fit After Thirty-Five With Jimmy Connors*.

Dr. Gordon is a member of the American Heart Association and American Diabetes Association. He is a fellow of the American College of Sports Medicine and the American Association of Cardiovascular and Pulmonary Rehabilitation (AACVPR). He has also served on the board of directors for AACVPR, the Texas Association of Cardiovascular and Pulmonary Rehabilitation, and the American Heart Association (Dallas affiliate).

Preface

A ny series of books as comprehensive as The Cooper Clinic and Research Institute Fitness Series is likely to have an interesting story behind it, and this one certainly does. The story began over a decade ago, shortly after I completed my medical training. Because of my keen interest in sports medicine (which was why I went to medical school in the first place), I volunteered to help establish an exercise rehabilitation program for my patients with chronic diseases at a major South African hospital. To get the ball rolling I decided to telephone patients who had recently been treated at the hospital. My very first call planted the seed for writing a series of books that would educate patients with chronic medical conditions about the many benefits of a physically active lifestyle and lead them step-by-step down the road to improved health.

That telephone call was an eye-opener for me, a relative novice in the field of rehabilitation medicine. The patient, a middle-aged man who had recently suffered from a heart attack, bellowed into the phone: "Why are you trying to create more problems for me? Isn't it enough that I've been turned into an invalid for the rest of my life by a heart attack?" Fortunately I kept my cool and convinced him to give the program a try—after all, what did he have to lose? Within months he was "miraculously" transformed into a man with a new zest for life. Like the thousands of men and women with chronic disorders with whom I've subsequently worked in South Africa and, more recently, the United States, he had experienced first-hand the numerous physical and psychological benefits of a medically prescribed exercise rehabilitation program.

Today it's known that a comprehensive exercise rehabilitation program, such as the one outlined in this book, is an essential component of state-of-the-art medical care for patients with a variety of chronic conditions (including stroke). But despite the many benefits unfolding through numerous research studies, patients with chronic medical conditions are usually not much better informed than that heart patient was prior to my telephone call. This book is meant to help fill this void for persons who have had a stroke by providing you with practical, easy-to-follow information about exercise rehabilitation for use in collaboration with your doctor.

To accomplish this, I've set out this book as follows. In chapter 1 you'll meet two of our stroke patients whose stories will introduce you to some basic concepts about strokes, exercise, and rehabilitation. In chapter 2 you'll discover the wonderful benefits of a physically active lifestyle. Toward the end of this chapter, however, I try to temper my obvious enthusiasm for exercise by pointing out some of its potential risks. In chapter 3 I'll show you step-by-step how to embark on a sensible exercise rehabilitation program. In chapter 4 you'll learn how to use the Health Points System to determine precisely how much exercise you need to do to optimize your health and fitness, without exerting yourself to the point where exercise can become risky. At the end of this chapter, I'll give you some useful tips for sticking with your exercise program once you get started. Finally, in chapter 5 I'll provide you with essential safety guidelines. Although exercise is a far more normal state for the human body than being sedentary, I want you to keep your risk, however small it may be, as low as possible.

View the programs in this book as prototypes. It is up to you and your doctor to make changes in these prototypes—that is, to adapt my programs—to suit the medical realities of your specific case. Set realistic goals for yourself. Above all, remember that no book can remove the need for close supervision by a patient's own doctor.

By the time you have completed this book, I hope that you'll have renewed hope for a healthier, longer, more enjoyable life. If you then act on the advice and adopt a more physically active lifestyle, this book will have supplemented the efforts of the National

Stroke Association in the United States, the American Heart Association, and other similar organizations around the world in the battle against stroke. If it does, the time spent preparing *Stroke: Your Complete Exercise Guide* will have been well worth the effort.

Neil F. Gordon, MD, PhD, MPH

Acknowledgments

To prepare a series of books as comprehensive and complex as this, I have required the assistance and cooperation of many talented people. To adequately acknowledge all would be impossible. However, I would be remiss not to recognize a few special contributions.

Ken Cooper, MD, MPH, chairman and founder of the Cooper Clinic, was of immense assistance in initiating this series. In addition to writing the foreword and providing many useful suggestions, he continues to serve as an inspiration to me and millions of people around the world.

Larry Gibbons, MD, MPH, medical director of the Cooper Clinic, co-authored with me *The Cooper Clinic Cardiac Rehabilitation Program*. In doing so he made an invaluable contribution to many of the concepts used in this series, especially the Health Points System.

Jacqueline Thompson, a talented writer based in Staten Island, New York, provided excellent editorial assistance with the first draft of this series. Her contributions and those of Herb Katz, a New York-based literary agent, greatly enhanced the practical value of this series.

Charles Sterling, EdD, executive director of The Cooper Institute for Aerobics Research, provided much needed guidance and support while working on this series. So too did John Duncan, PhD, Chris Scott, MS, Pat Brill, PhD, Kia Vaandrager, MS, Conrad Earnest, MS,

Sheila Burford, and my many other colleagues at the Institute, Cooper Clinic, Cooper Wellness Program, and Cooper Fitness Center.

John Basmajian, MD, a world-renowned stroke authority from McMaster University, Canada, reviewed the first draft of *Stroke: Your Complete Exercise Guide* and provided many excellent suggestions.

My thanks to Rainer Martens, president of Human Kinetics Publishers, without whom this series could not have been published. Rainer, Holly Gilly (my developmental editor), and other staff members at Human Kinetics Publishers did a fantastic job in making this series a reality. It was a pleasurable and gratifying experience to work with them.

A special thanks to the patients who allowed me to tell their stories and to all my patients over the years from whom I have learned so much about exercise and rehabilitation.

Finally I want to thank my wonderful family—my wife, Tracey, and daughters, Kim and Terri—for their patience, support, and understanding in preparing this series.

To these people, and the many others far too numerous to list, many thanks for making this book a reality and in so doing benefiting stroke patients around the world.

Credits

Developmental Editor—Holly Gilly; *Assistant Editors*—Valerie Hall, Dawn Roselund, Julie Swadener; *Copyeditor*—Jane Bowers; *Proofreader*—Julia Anderson; *Indexer*—Theresa J. Schaeffer; *Production Director*—Ernie Noa; *Text Design*—Keith Blomberg; *Text Layout*—Angela K. Snyder, Tara Welsch; *Cover Design*—Jack Davis; *Factoids*—Doug Burnett; *Technique Drawings*—Tim Offenstein; *Interior Art*—Kathy Fuoss, Gretchen Walters; *Printer*—United Graphics

The Cooper Clinic and Research Institute Fitness Series

Arthritis: *Your Complete Exercise Guide*

Breathing Disorders: *Your Complete Exercise Guide*

Chronic Fatigue: *Your Complete Exercise Guide*

Diabetes: *Your Complete Exercise Guide*

Stroke: *Your Complete Exercise Guide*

Chapter 1

Moving Beyond
the Disability
of a Stroke

You've had a stroke. Be thankful you're alive. Be thankful, as well, that you had your stroke recently and not 50 years ago, when effective treatment and rehabilitation for this condition were almost nonexistent. The case of Franklin Delano Roosevelt, the 32nd president of the United States, illustrates the impotence of earlier medical authorities in dealing with high blood pressure and stroke.[1]

A person who has uncontrolled high blood pressure, or *hypertension*, is a prime candidate for a stroke, as you no doubt know. Roosevelt's doctors knew it too but were powerless to do much about it. Here's a capsule medical history of what happened to Roosevelt between 1933 when he assumed office and his death three terms later in 1945.

Roosevelt's blood pressure was normal (136/78*) during his first few years in office. By 1937, it was inching up, although at this stage

---

*The first figure represents the systolic blood pressure, the pressure exerted on the walls of the arteries when the heart contracts, forcing blood out to all parts of the body. The second figure represents the diastolic blood pressure exerted between heartbeats when the cardiovascular system takes a tiny rest. The medical definition of hypertension is systolic blood pressure equal to or greater than 140 mmHg or diastolic blood pressure equal to or greater than 90 mmHg, or both.

there was no apparent damage to his heart, kidneys, or other vital organs and certainly no symptoms. Nobody was terribly concerned.

Roosevelt's condition progressed relentlessly—from 162/98 in 1937 to 188/105 in 1944. His doctors knew that his condition was becoming increasingly dangerous. In fact, just before his fatal stroke, they had detected evidence of heart enlargement. Their not-very-effective remedy—the standard treatment back then—was a low-fat diet, massages to ease tension and stress, and regular doses of pheno-barbital, a mild sedative.

By early 1945, with his blood pressure vacillating between 180/110 and 230/130, Roosevelt's disorder had worsened to the point where he had to sleep upright in a chair because when he lay prone, his lungs would accumulate fluid as a result of heart failure, seriously hampering his breathing. Those famous photos of Roosevelt with Churchill and Stalin at the Yalta Conference were telling, indeed. Roosevelt had circles under his eyes and looked drawn and wan. He was sleeping only 3 or 4 hours a night, he suffered from headaches, and he was showing symptoms of heart failure. On April 12, 1945, at the age of only 63, he had a massive stroke and died within the hour.

Today, with the wide array of targeted treatments to manage high blood pressure, most people are more fortunate than Roosevelt: They bypass stroke entirely. Those who do have one usually survive and are eventually rehabilitated to where they can get around on their own. And with proper care, the risk of a follow-up stroke is minimized.

Provided you've progressed to where any stroke-related paralysis has largely disappeared, I think you'll find that the exercise rehabilitation program outlined in this book offers one of your best hopes for staying energetic and involved in life. Indeed, it's regular exercise at The Cooper Aerobics Center that's partly responsible for the slow but steady recuperation of the man and near-miraculous recovery of the woman you're about to meet.

CASE HISTORY OF ROGER KNIGHT

Roger Knight, a retired accountant, was 67 when he had his stroke. Before his stroke, Roger's looks betrayed that he wasn't in the peak of health. He was overweight, seldom exercised, and seemed somewhat older than his years. For a man his age, there was no spring to his step, no enthusiastic engagement with life.

Roger's medical episode began when he went to his doctor for an annual checkup before a trip to Europe. Technically, his condition was

OK with a few notable exceptions: His blood pressure was mildly elevated (164/98), and his electrocardiogram (ECG) suggested that his heart muscle might be thicker than it should be. His doctor ascribed the latter, a heart abnormality that can be a precursor of stroke, to his mild hypertension. He pointed out that Roger would have to get serious about lowering his blood pressure as soon as he returned from this vacation.

But Roger's condition worsened faster than expected. While in Europe, on two occasions Roger had 10-minute episodes in which he suddenly lost his balance, had blurred vision, and felt his left arm and leg become noticeably weak. Roger blamed the episodes on the excitement of sight-seeing and being places he'd read about for years, but his wife, Liz, was concerned.

As Roger later learned, the spells that he viewed as harmless were warning signs of an impending stroke. The spells were *transient ischemic attacks* (TIAs). Someone who has had a TIA is 13 times more likely than others to have a stroke sometime in the next year. In Roger's case, the time interval was telescoped. Three days after he returned home, Roger had a stroke. It damaged the right side of his brain, leaving his left arm and leg partly paralyzed. The doctor referred to Roger's impaired condition as *hemiplegia*, meaning the paralysis affected only one side of his body.

To his credit, Roger was never a man to let adversity pin him down. To his wife's enormous relief, he was a model patient, following all the instructions and suggestions of his physician and the other members of his health-care team. Thanks to intensive rehabilitation and eager family support, Roger was about 60% back to normal within 3 months of his near-fatal cerebral event. He could walk, albeit with a walker, and was reinvolved in family financial affairs and other matters. Over the next few months he continued to get better as he applied the things he learned as a member of the National Stroke Association. (For information about the association and its many outstanding services, write to National Stroke Association, 300 E. Hampden Ave., Suite 240, Englewood, CO 80110-2654, USA.) He never missed the NSA's local chapter meetings or a session of his stroke support group.

But despite his great recuperative strides, Roger was depressed and dissatisfied with his progress. His brush with the medical community and an exposure to the whole notion of preventive health care had piqued his curiosity. For the first time in his life, he was reading newspaper health columns, borrowing health books from the library, and scrutinizing what was on his plate at mealtimes. Gradually, the notion crystallized that simply feeling all right again wasn't good enough. He wanted to feel exceptional, to be more functional, agile,

Case history, Roger Knight

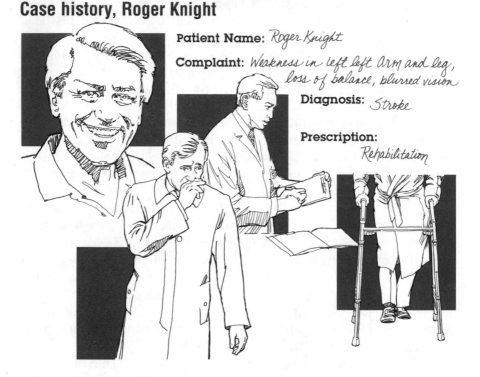

Patient Name: *Roger Knight*

Complaint: *Weakness in left left arm and leg, loss of balance, blurred vision*

Diagnosis: *Stroke*

Prescription:
Rehabilitation

and energized than before his stroke. In short, he wanted to turn back the clock and grow younger.

A year after his stroke, it was this goal that led Roger to the Cooper Clinic for further medical and nutritional advice, and he joined The Cooper Aerobics Center as a regular exerciser. Roger's major remaining disabilities were difficulty in climbing stairs without holding onto a rail, muscular weakness, low stamina, and a tendency to tire too easily. He had what I'd categorize as a slight disability.

I explained to Roger that regular exercise would have little value in reversing any neurological impairments; most of that reversal had taken place during his first 6 months of rehabilitation. But exercise could help alleviate some of the functional disability caused by such impairments. It could almost certainly erase much of his easy fatigability and lack of strength. Moreover, it could help reduce his risk of ever having another stroke or a heart attack. (As I have mentioned, heart disease is a related cardiovascular malady that stroke survivors have to be extremely careful about.)

I also suggested that Roger might be more successful in adopting the exercise habit long-term if his wife became involved so they could eventually work out together and bolster each other's resolve. Liz was more than happy to oblige if it would help Roger. (She seemed to disregard the fact that in the process she'd be boosting her own chances of living a longer, healthier life.)

At first, the couple worked out separately, because Roger needed to begin with 12 weeks of exercise skill-building in our medically supervised program. The treadmill exercise test that every rehabilitation patient undergoes indicated that Roger's fitness level was poor, so I started him off very, very slowly. During the first week, all he did was gentle range-of-motion and stretching exercises, some muscle strengthening, and an easy walk around our indoor rubberized track. By Week 2, he was ready to augment the 2-1/2 minutes of daily walking with a second 2-1/2 minutes of stationary cycling on a bike that worked both his arms and legs. Each week, Roger added 2-1/2 minutes to his walks and to his bike workouts until, by Week 10, he was up to 45 minutes of aerobic exercise (walking and/or cycling) 3 days a week.

Because frequent fatigue continued to trouble Roger, I suggested he try interval training. This involves replacing one long, endurance-oriented workout with a series of shorter exercise bouts, each separated by a brief rest period. For example, rather than cycling for 20 minutes without stopping, Roger would divide his ride into four mini-sessions. He'd cycle for 5-minute periods with 1 minute at a very low intensity in between. If he was really fatigued, he would rest completely for a minute or so, although I explained that low-intensity cycling is always preferable. (An abrupt cessation of exertion is not a good idea, as I'll discuss when I cover warm-up and cool-down in chapter 5.)

After 12 weeks, many patients are ready to start exercising without a qualified health-care professional standing by, but Roger wasn't one of them. During the next 3 months, Roger kept track of his exertion using our Health Points System. Goaded by this incentive, Roger, a retired accountant, seemed to draw strength from tallying the numbers each day. Suddenly he began to advance faster; by the end of 6 months of supervised exercise, he was earning 50 health points a week, our minimum recommended goal.

For the last 6 months, Roger has been working out on his own. He's been exercising when he wants and where he wants, but he continues to abide by my special safety guidelines for stroke patients. Today, he consistently earns the recommended 50 to 100 health points a week. His progress shows in his fitness level, which has increased 45% since he started his program a year ago. His strength has grown by 70%. His wife is pleased with his new physique—he's lost 30 pounds and is slim and trim. Roger tells me he feels 100% better and that his self-image has improved. Best of all, his doctor recently announced that Roger could reduce the dosage of his blood-pressure medication.

Liz, who works out with Roger at the center 3 days a week, has her own success story. But she says the most important change for both of them is the beneficial impact that working toward the common goal of better health has had on their marriage.

KO GREEN: COMEBACK-OF-THE-YEAR AWARD WINNER

Roger's story is one of incremental improvement over an extended period. Ko Green's recovery, on the other hand, is an example of steely determination and grit that paid off far faster—and more completely—than anyone predicted. In fact, the 9-hour surgery to locate the aneurysm that had triggered Ko's stroke was so risky that doctors later admitted she only had a 20-to-1 shot at survival. But live to tell the tale she certainly has. At a Cooper Aerobics Center banquet a year or so after her stroke, we gave Ko an award for achieving the most remarkable recovery most of us had ever witnessed.[2]

Unlike Roger, Ko, at 49, was physically fit and had no hypertension, weight problem, or craving for unhealthy foods. She was a 25-year veteran of the running track and enjoyed other sports as well. One of them was skiing, and it was while on vacation in Colorado that she had a *hemorrhagic* stroke, a different type of stroke entirely than Roger had, one with no warning signs. The cause was a ruptured blood vessel at the base of Ko's brain. It happened because of a blood-vessel defect no one could have known about.

Ko's neurological impairments were extensive. After surgery, her throat and right arm and leg were partly paralyzed, and one eyeball was turned around in the socket so that the white part was all that was visible. "I drooled all the time," she recalled, "and I could hardly speak. The whole experience seemed like a bad dream where my memory had gone fuzzy."

Ko's excellent cardiovascular conditioning was a prime factor in her survival. All those years of exercise seemed to give her an instinctive knowledge about how to fight her disabilities.

On the way out of the hospital, Ko insisted on getting out of her wheelchair and hobbling through the lobby door. Every day thereafter, via indecipherable grunts and sign language, she'd "commandeer"

Case history, Ko Green

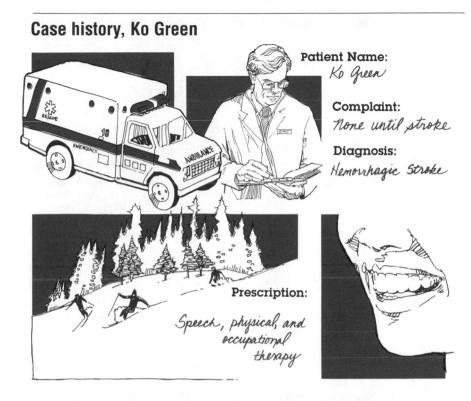

Patient Name:
Ko Green

Complaint:
None until stroke

Diagnosis:
Hemorrhagic Stroke

Prescription:
Speech, physical, and occupational therapy

someone to help her take a walk around the block. She also worked regularly with speech, physical, and occupational therapists.

Within 4 months, Ko had improved enough (to her health-care team's utter amazement) to visit The Cooper Aerobics Center. With her nurse standing on the sidelines and frowning, Ko's first stab at formal exercise was a basic calisthenics and stretching class. She stayed in the back row and did what she could, which at first was mainly lifting her left leg. "My nurse felt I was doing too much, but I guess she had a grudging respect for my determination," Ko said.

Over the next 5 months, Ko logged 137 miles of walking and jogging around the paths winding through our property. Soon she started to jog in earnest and drive a car. And as soon as she was physically able to, Ko began coming to The Cooper Aerobics Center every weekday morning to jog 3 to 5 miles and take an exercise class. Eventually Ko was once again enjoying 10K fun-runs.

When asked how she felt then, Ko replied, "I feel good. I feel normal, although I still have trouble with my memory sometimes. You can't imagine how much I appreciate running now because, for a long while, I never thought I'd ever do it again. That's what makes it so special."

WHAT IS A STROKE?

A stroke is a potentially fatal cutoff of the blood supply to part of the brain. No part of the body can survive an interruption in its blood supply for long because blood dispenses life-sustaining oxygen and other fuels, but the brain is especially vulnerable. The brain, after all, is the control center of the body, directing every thought and physical action. When there's a malfunction in the brain, it shows up in a person's behavior and actions, or lack thereof, almost immediately.

There are two broad categories of stroke: ischemic strokes, such as Roger experienced, and strokes due to a surprise hemorrhage, like the one Ko Green had.[3] About 82% of strokes are ischemic. Although hemorrhagic strokes are less common, they are also more deadly.[4]

Ischemic Strokes

When the blood supply to any part of the brain is reduced, brain *ischemia* develops and the oxygen-starved cells in that area stop functioning properly. Whether they stop working temporarily or die depends on the degree of ischemia and its duration.

Milder ischemic spells, or TIAs, such as the two Roger had on his vacation, cause the brain cells to pause in their normal functioning for usually a matter of minutes, to at most 24 hours. Once an adequate amount of nourishing blood starts coursing through vessels again, those cells begin to revive and bodily functions are shortly restored. More severe ischemia that lasts longer ultimately crosses over some invisible boundary line and becomes what's known as a stroke, or a *cerebrovascular accident* (CVA). An *ischemic stroke* is an extreme form of ischemia that causes irreversible death of brain cells, known as brain *infarction*.

The cause of ischemic strokes is similar to that of heart disease. Fatty deposits called *atherosclerotic plaques* are usually the culprits in both conditions, but the plaque buildup that causes ischemic stroke is on the inside walls of the arteries in the neck and head instead of the coronary arteries leading to the heart. Atherosclerotic plaques can cause a stroke by completely blocking off an artery leading to the brain. But it's more common for plaques simply to narrow the artery, making the blood flow more turbulent and instigating the formation of a blood clot, or *thrombus*. A thrombus that forms in a narrowed arterial passage can act like a plug, stopping blood flow and precipitating a stroke. Or a fragment of a thrombus—called an *embolus* or wandering blood clot—can break off and get stuck in one of the smaller blood vessels in the brain. A person with heart disease is at increased risk for a stroke because there's always the threat that an embolus emanating from a malfunctioning heart can travel via the bloodstream and lodge itself in the brain.

Hemorrhagic Strokes

The second category of stroke is triggered by a hemorrhage. A hemorrhage can occur anywhere in the body, but a hemorrhage in or around the brain is a life-and-death matter. A hemorrhagic stroke occurs when an artery leading to the brain bursts, spilling blood into the brain or into the cavity between the outer surface of the brain and the skull. There are several causes of hemorrhagic strokes. In Ko Green's case, unbeknownst to her, she had a weak spot in her arterial wall, possibly inherited, called an *aneurysm*. Burst aneurysms are a relatively common cause of hemorrhagic strokes. Hemorrhagic strokes also typically occur in people who have both atherosclerosis and high blood pressure. So to a certain extent, people can reduce their chances of such a stroke by living a healthier lifestyle.

Hemorrhagic strokes are far more likely to be fatal. Not only may they disrupt the blood flow to the part of the brain where the burst artery leads, but they place pressure on the brain and cause brain tissue to swell. Should a person survive such a stroke, the pressure and swelling in the brain may subside spontaneously over time. Or, as was the situation with Ko Green, surgery may be needed to relieve the pressure and swelling. Survivors of such operations often recover fully or close to fully.

Although the survival rate is higher for ischemic strokes than for hemorrhagic strokes, the resultant neurological impairment from ischemic stroke can be more severe and recovery less assured.

NEUROLOGICAL IMPAIRMENT AND THE THREE PHASES OF STROKE RECOVERY

No two strokes are exactly alike because several factors influence the outcome. They include the type of stroke, the extent of the brain damage, and, most importantly, where the damage occurs, because certain regions of the brain control specific body functions.

Figure 1.1 shows how the site of brain injury influences the kind of neurological impairments a stroke survivor experiences. As the figure makes clear, there's a cross-over effect. Paralysis of the *right side of the body* (referred to as *right hemiplegia*) occurs when the stroke has damaged part of the *left side of the brain*, and vice versa. Typically, people with left brain damage will also have difficulty with speech and language. Also, their behavior is altered. They're somewhat cautious, anxious, and disorganized when attempting new tasks.

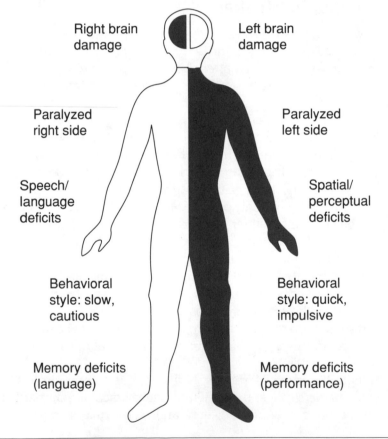

Right brain damage

Left brain damage

Paralyzed right side

Paralyzed left side

Speech/ language deficits

Spatial/ perceptual deficits

Behavioral style: slow, cautious

Behavioral style: quick, impulsive

Memory deficits (language)

Memory deficits (performance)

Figure 1.1   The effects of a stroke. Trace the shading in the drawing of this stroke patient from one side of the brain to the opposite side of the body. Right brain damage causes the disabilities listed on the left side of the body. In contrast, left brain damage causes the disabilities listed on the right side of the body.

Adaptation reproduced with permission. "How Stroke Affects Behavior," 1992. Copyright American Heart Association.

In contrast, people with left hemiplegia (paralysis of the left side of the body due to right brain damage) have spatial-perceptual deficits, or an impaired ability to judge distance, size, position, speed of movement, form, and the relation of parts to wholes. Such people give a false sense of nondisability because they tend to talk better than they are actually able to perform. They may also be impulsive and careless.

Stroke has been studied enough that certain generalizations can be made about the recovery process. The phases of recovery are described as follows:[5]

Within a few hours to several months after a stroke, many patients gradually experience a partial or even complete reversal of their neurological impairments—for example, their paralysis, loss of sensation, and confused mental state. The purpose of a formal rehabilitation program is to assist in and accelerate this recovery process. The body is most receptive to the beneficial impact of physical and other rehabilitative therapies during the first 6 months after a stroke, so that's when a concentrated effort is usually made to reverse the neurological malfunctioning and, in so doing, eliminate disability. The patient and family members work closely with a stroke rehabilitation team of physicians; specially trained nurses; physical, occupational, and speech therapists; and social workers.

Phases of the recovery process

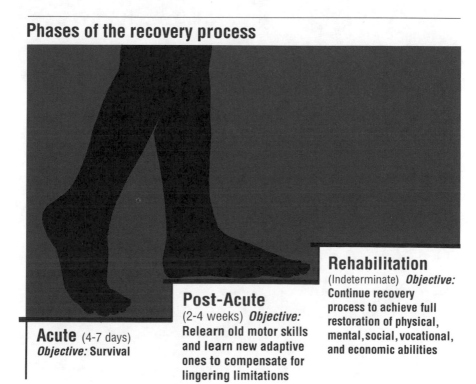

Acute (4-7 days)
Objective: Survival

Post-Acute
(2-4 weeks) *Objective:* Relearn old motor skills and learn new adaptive ones to compensate for lingering limitations

Rehabilitation
(Indeterminate) *Objective:* Continue recovery process to achieve full restoration of physical, mental, social, vocational, and economic abilities

But the restoration of function doesn't abruptly stop at the 6-month point. Quite the contrary. It tends to continue, in abated form, for up to 2 years after a stroke.[3] During this time (and even at a later stage), it's still possible to reduce the degree of disability that results from neurological malfunctioning. For example, although you may always walk with a limp due to an irreversible neurological impairment, you may still be able to increase the distance you can walk and, thus, reduce your degree of disability. That's why I want to encourage those of you who've made it to the mild- or moderate-disability stage within 6 months or so to use the exercise program in this book to continue your improvement. Carefully orchestrated exercise, following my special safety guidelines for stroke patients, should help you overcome some of the lingering disability you still have.[6]

If you've survived a stroke, you have reason to be hopeful about the future. A Rochester, MN, study of stroke survivors at the 6-month point revealed that 27% have no lingering physical disability, 24% have slight disability, 23% have moderate disability, 11% have a more significant disability, and only 6% are severely disabled.[7] These are the categories of the well-known Rankin Disability Scale discussed in the next chapter.

Chapter 2

The Benefits and Risks of Exercise for Stroke Recovery and Prevention

It's a sad fact that most stroke patients stop exercising once their formal rehabilitation program ends. They reason that 6 months or so of therapy has erased as much of the neurological impairment as possible,[1,2] so why continue exercise when little obvious benefit will be forthcoming?

REDUCES DEGREE OF DISABILITY

This thinking is out-of-date and ignores what investigators have discovered about exercise and stroke in recent years. First, I must reemphasize that although you can expect little turnaround in *neurological function* after the first 6 months, exercise rehabilitation performed after this time can still help reduce a person's *degree of disability*. This is attested to by a recent study conducted by physical therapists from Pacific University in Oregon. They evaluated the changes that 1 month of intensive rehabilitation, including physical exercise, had on the functional capacities of stroke patients who were at least 1 year removed from their strokes. The results were positive. The therapists discovered that significant improvements could still be fostered at this late date. The study participants made noticeable headway in their ability to perform the many activities of daily living, things that other people take for granted.[3]

INCREASES PHYSICAL FITNESS

The one benefit of long-term, regular exercise that can almost always be guaranteed—even in elderly patients and those with chronic conditions such as heart and brain disorders—is an increase in physical fitness.[4,5] With a higher fitness level, you can exert yourself more strenuously for longer periods of time. With more energy, you'll have more reserve for participating in new activities—or in old ones that you mistakenly thought you didn't care about anymore. The result is an increase in functional capacity and a decrease in disability.[6]

REDUCES THE CHANCES OF
A SECOND STROKE

In addition to reducing disability and increasing fitness, a third key fact to remember as you consider an exercise program is this: Moderate exertion several days a week is likely to greatly reduce the chances that you'll develop a second stroke or die prematurely from other potentially fatal chronic diseases.

Stroke is a recurrent disease. Because you've had one stroke, you're five times more likely to have other ones. Put another way, 62% of people who have a stroke survive it; about one quarter of stroke survivors can expect to have a second stroke unless they do something positive to prevent it.[7] Regular exercise is now believed to be one way to reduce that risk significantly.[8] This is one of the primary reasons you should start exercising once your formal stroke rehabilitation program is over—that is, if you can.

I qualified that last statement because not every stroke survivor recovers to the point of being able to undertake my exercise program. The following box shows the Rankin Disability Scale. Disabilities in Grades 1 to 3 generally won't keep you from exercising, although people with Grade 3 disabilities often need close supervision by a health-care professional. The exercise program I outline is probably out of the question for people with Grade 4 disabilities and definitely for those with Grade 5.

RANKIN STROKE DISABILITY SCALE

Grade 1 Disability
(none or almost none)

You're able to carry out all your usual tasks and duties.

Grade 2 Disability
(slight)

You're no longer able to do some previous activities, but you can look after yourself and your own affairs without assistance.

Grade 3 Disability
(moderate)

You require some help, but you're able to walk without the assistance of another person, although you may use a cane.

Grade 4 Disability
(moderately severe)

You're unable to walk without assistance from another person. You need someone's help to accomplish most self-care activities such as bathing, going to the toilet, grooming, etc.

Grade 5 Disability
(severe)

You're bedridden and incontinent, and you require constant nursing care and attention.

Note: From "Cerebral Vascular Accidents in Patients Over the Age of 60: II. Prognosis." J. Rankin, 1957, *Scottish Medical Journal*, **2**, 200-215. Adapted by permission.

Large-scale studies on stroke tend to concentrate on how to prevent a first stroke. Many such investigations pinpoint a lack of exercise (a sedentary lifestyle, in other words) as an important factor predisposing someone to a stroke.[9-13] For example, in a recent study conducted at The Cooper Institute for Aerobics Research, 11,973 initially healthy Cooper Clinic patients were followed for an average of 8 years. Those who were not physically fit were about three times more likely to have a stroke than the physically fit study subjects.[14, 15]

What does the medical literature say about follow-up strokes? Medical investigators to date haven't probed that question, at least not directly. But something is known about what stroke survivors eventually die from. Some die from another stroke, but far more die from coronary heart disease, a closely allied problem.[16] This is hardly surprising because stroke and coronary heart disease often have the same underlying cause: a dangerous buildup of atherosclerotic plaques. The buildup is just in different arteries, although plaque accumulation often takes place simultaneously at various sites. In fact, atherosclerosis of the head and neck arteries is often accompanied by significant atherosclerosis in the coronary arteries leading to the heart—one reason why people with heart disease often have strokes (and stroke survivors often have heart disease).

REDUCES THE RISK OF DYING FROM CARDIOVASCULAR DISEASE

There's ample evidence that regular exercise can reduce the risk of dying from coronary heart disease by almost 50% in people who've never had a heart attack, and by 25% in people who have.[17,18] Specific studies have not probed the efficacy of exercise in stroke survivors, but I think it's logical to apply such heart disease statistics to people who have had a stroke. After all, the origins, development, and eventual outcomes of the two health problems are so closely intertwined.

Just as is the case with heart attacks, ischemic strokes (and hemorrhagic ones that are due to the combination of atherosclerosis and hypertension) can be predicted to a certain extent. This is because medical researchers have isolated the preconditions that make such strokes more likely. Many of these risk factors are the same as those for coronary heart disease. Today the medical community is more concerned about preventive medicine and places a great deal of emphasis on modification of stroke patients' risk factors, the first step in preventing a follow-up stroke.[2,19]

The stroke risk factors highlighted in the following box are ones that exercise can help reverse, or even eliminate. They are important risk factors, so you should do anything you can to alter them for the better. *This is another reason you should take exercise seriously.*

STROKE RISK FACTORS THAT REGULAR EXERCISE CAN INFLUENCE FOR THE BETTER

You can expect a regular exercise program to have a positive impact on all the stroke risk factors I list below. On the other hand, exercise has no impact on some other stroke risk factors— with two possible exceptions: Strenuous exercise has on rare occasions been known to have a harmful effect in people who suffer from sickle cell disease or who, like Ko Green, have un- treated (indeed, unsuspected) blood vessel structural deficiencies, such as aneurysms.

Lifestyle Risk Factors

- Cigarette smoking. Studies show that people who exercise are more likely to stop smoking—permanently. Also, regular exercise helps offset some of the negative effects of ciga- rette smoking.
- Drug abuse.
- Type A personality.
- Sedentary way of life.
- Obesity.
- Abnormal blood cholesterol and lipoproteins.

Disease Risk Factors

- High blood pressure.
- Coronary heart disease and certain other cardiac diseases.
- Atherosclerosis of the head and neck arteries.
- Blood-component imbalance. Too high a concentration of red blood cells for a given amount of fluid, or *plasma*, in the blood predisposes a person to blood-clot formation.
- Diabetes.

Source: Adapted from National Institute of Neurological Disorders and Stroke, "Classifi- cation of Cerebrovascular Diseases III." *Stroke*, 21 (1990): 637-676.

High blood pressure heads the lineup of disease risk factors. Persis- tent hypertension is widely regarded as the quintessential risk factor for stroke.

Recently, my colleagues and I examined what people with high blood pressure can do to lower their blood pressure levels *without taking drugs.* We considered these possibilities: do regular aerobic exercise; lose weight; cut down on salt in the diet; increase potassium intake; practice biofeedback; and pursue relaxation therapy. We reviewed the available studies and found that after shedding pounds (if a person is overweight), aerobic exercise is the most effective nondrug treatment for hypertension. Next comes relaxation therapy.[20]

When you exercise, you burn up calories; this obviously helps foster weight loss. So, for reducing hypertension, aerobic exercise actually has a two-fold effect: not only does it help lower blood pressure directly, it also helps lower it indirectly by aiding in weight loss.[21]

MAKES LIFE MORE WORTH LIVING

Most stroke survivors experience a relatively good recovery during the initial months of formal rehabilitation, but (as I know from my own experience and that of other physicians) the overall quality of life for nonexercising stroke patients seldom returns to prestroke levels. This is what one patient, whom I'll call Joe, told me in a moment of candor just before he became a regular at The Cooper Aerobics Center. Our staff conducts lengthy interviews with all our new stroke patients, and Joe's comments are typical:

> Sure, I've reached the point where I can take care of my needs again. I'm independent. I can function at home and, to some extent, at work. I don't have a bum arm and leg anymore. I no longer slur my words. I can think more or less coherently most of the time. But am I back to where I was before I was stricken? Of course not. When I had the stroke, I took a giant step backwards and I've only moved forward again part of the way.

What Joe had to say is borne out in studies, especially a recent one in Helsinki, Finland. It involved a group of stroke survivors, all under 65 years old, who were queried about their abilities and overall outlook 4 years after their strokes. Some 87% of them had long since recovered to the point where they were independent and almost completely free of disabilities. The following figure shows how these people felt about life after a stroke.[22]

This isn't the only study to report such sad tidings about the emotional aftermath of stroke. Other researchers have reported similar findings.[23]

Once again, because no exercise studies have specifically targeted stroke survivors, what I'm about to say is based on the anecdotal

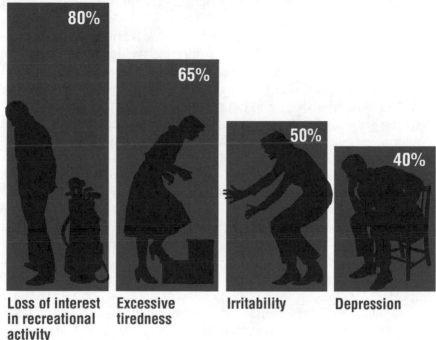

Feelings of stroke survivors 4 years later

- 80% — **Loss of interest in recreational activity**
- 65% — **Excessive tiredness**
- 50% — **Irritability**
- 40% — **Depression**

evidence I've garnered in my experiences working with stroke patients and from inferences that can be made from studies with heart attack survivors.

Psychological and Emotional Benefits

It's well known, and indisputable, that exercise brings about many physiological benefits. It's somewhat less well known, but also documented in the medical literature, that exercise can confer psychological and emotional benefits.

Joe is a perfect example. He was mildly depressed when he began his exercise program. At first, he complained a lot about the small disabilities he still had and was grumpy when I tried to get him to see the brighter side of his situation. Slowly, over the first 12 weeks of his supervised exercise effort, Joe's outlook began to change. For one thing, coming to The Cooper Aerobics Center several days a week to work out with his peers gave him something to look forward to. He began to feel less worn-out and tired all the time. But the real breakthrough in his mood came when he realized how much more energy he now had to pursue the hobbies and interests he'd dropped after his stroke.

I'd be foolish to claim that regular exercise is a panacea for psychological problems, but based on scientific as well as such anecdotal evidence, I do know it can help profoundly. Several studies have concluded that people with chronic diseases who exercise regularly have less stress, anxiety, and depression; they sleep better; and they have an enhanced sense of self-esteem.[24] A consensus panel of the National Institute of Mental Health in the United States likewise maintains that exercise and physical fitness have a positive influence on most people's mental outlook and well-being, regardless of age. Regular exercise helps control stress, reduce anxiety, and meliorate depression. Although major depression requires medication and psychotherapy, exercise is seen as a useful adjunct to them (remember that the combination of some drugs and exercise requires close medical monitoring).[25]

The role exercise can play in overcoming depression is especially important for stroke survivors. Not only is depression common among them, but it's well documented that such a negative state often makes them, temporarily and intermittently, give up on life. A depressed stroke patient has less willpower or determination to be self-reliant and overcome any remaining disabilities.[26, 27]

Improves Self-Esteem

How can participation in an exercise program enhance self-esteem? About 50% of people who start an exercise program drop out within 3 to 6 months. If you can defy this statistic, imagine how you'll feel. Exercise will come to symbolize your perseverance, your ability to make a commitment and stick with it. Exercise will provide tangible proof that you really do have more control than you thought over your condition. This knowledge will help prevent a syndrome known as *learned helplessness,* in which patients believe their disability is beyond their control, to be borne with as much stoicism as possible. Learned helplessness results in a vicious downward spiral of further psychological problems and dependence on others. Taken to its logical conclusion, invalidism is the result.

Ken Cooper likes to tout exercise as "nature's own tranquilizer." He and others believe that this tranquilizing effect occurs in part because endurance exercise triggers the release of endorphins, hormones produced by the pituitary gland in the brain. Once endorphins enter the bloodstream, their beneficial effects are thought to last 2 or 3 hours. Among those effects is a sense of euphoria, a feeling that all is right with the world.

By now I hope I've convinced you of the many benefits of a physically active lifestyle for persons who have had a stroke. But please keep in mind that exercise is not a panacea but an important supplemental therapy. To be most effective, regular exercise must be combined with appropriate medical care as well as other positive lifestyle changes (stopping smoking and eating nutritiously, for example).

RISKS OF EXERCISE

Yes, there are some. The major health hazards of *vigorous* exercise for anyone, whether or not that person has had a stroke, are sudden death and musculoskeletal injuries. For you as a stroke survivor, there's the special risk that the wrong kind of exercise could be detrimental to your cerebrovascular condition or could worsen any other chronic diseases you may have.

Sudden Death During Exercise

You've probably read or heard about people who drop dead suddenly while exercising. It's a chilling picture, to be sure—one that might make you wonder if it's really safe to exercise, especially now that you've had a stroke.

Studies done at The Cooper Aerobics Center and elsewhere show that having a stroke while exercising is exceptionally rare—and dying suddenly from it while still in your exercise clothes is even rarer.[28-30] The occasional stroke that does occur during exercise is almost always of the hemorrhagic type.[31]

These studies indicate that the combination of injudicious, vigorous exertion and preexisting coronary heart disease accounts for most exercise-related deaths in adults. It's not simply exertion. In chapter 5, I'll explain how to determine whether you have coronary heart disease. I'll also tell you how to minimize your chances of having a potentially fatal cardiovascular event during exercise, be it another stroke or a heart attack. Be assured that when appropriate precautions are taken, exercise is likely to be exceptionally safe, even for you with your medical history.[32]

Musculoskeletal Injuries

It probably doesn't come as news to you that even healthy adults who exercise sustain musculoskeletal injuries occasionally. Two recent studies estimate that 50% of competitive runners sustain at least one exercise-related injury each year.[33, 34] But these are serious amateur or professional runners. When the sample involves only recreational exercisers, the story is much different. Such studies, including one conducted at The Cooper Institute for Aerobics Research,[35] suggest that the number of exercise-induced injuries among noncompetitive athletes is not nearly as high as popularly believed. In fact, it's estimated that musculoskeletal injuries serious enough to require medical care probably occur at an annual rate of less than 5% among recreational exercisers. (See chapter 3 for exercises that will help you prevent musculoskeletal injuries; they don't have to happen.)

Chapter 2

Prescription

❏ Include exercise in your stroke recovery and rehabilitation program.

❏ Exercise regularly to increase your functional capacity and minimize any disability caused by your stroke.

❏ Exercise regularly to reduce the chances that you'll have another stroke or die prematurely from another potentially fatal chronic disease.

❏ Exercise regularly to make life more worth living.

❏ Keep in mind that exercise is not a panacea but an important supplemental therapy.

❏ To gain optimal benefits, combine regular exercise with appropriate medical care and other positive lifestyle changes.

❏ Be aware that inappropriate exercise could be detrimental to your cardiovascular system or worsen other chronic diseases you may have.

❏ Obtain your doctor's consent before beginning an exercise program.

Chapter 3

Getting Started on a Regular Exercise Program

You might want to think of exercise as a form of medication. When you exercise, just as when you take a drug, you want to strike a balance between the two goals: effectiveness and safety. This chapter and the next will concentrate on effectiveness. I'll explain which types of exercise, and how much of each, you need to do for maximum health benefits. In chapter 5 I'll go on to discuss safety.

THE COMPONENTS OF AN EXERCISE WORKOUT

You should follow a sequence of activity in a typical exercise session: 10 to 20 minutes of stretching and muscle strengthening, 5 minutes of aerobic warm-up, 15 to 60 minutes of aerobic exercise at an appropriate intensity, 5 minutes of aerobic cool-down, and, finally, 5 minutes of stretching. (Keep in mind that it may take several weeks to work your way up to the durations of time I've specified.)

What's the rationale for doing all these forms of exercise? The aerobic portion of the workout, of course, is aimed squarely at reducing your risk for recurrent strokes and other chronic diseases, heart disease in particular. Yes, it's the most important. But range-of-motion exercises, stretching (or flexibility training), and muscle strengthening shouldn't be overlooked either. After all, without joints and muscles that function well, you can't undertake aerobics—and many other recreational, occupational, and self-care activities. Also, without strong, flexible muscles, you're more likely to experience a musculoskeletal injury. (Indeed, the strength and flexibility components of a balanced exercise program are so important that The Cooper Institute for Aerobics Research has recently written a book—*The Strength Connection*—that addresses them almost exclusively.[1] I am also conducting a 5-year study in this area with funds from the National Institute of Arthritis and Musculoskeletal and Skin Diseases.)

Range-of-Motion and Stretching Exercises

Range-of-motion and stretching exercises are part of a good exercise protocol. They should precede an aerobic exercise session, even if you are in good health and have never had a stroke. It won't take you long to appreciate the value of these exercises. They relax you mentally and physically, and they probably help prevent injuries by increasing your flexibility and widening your freedom of movement.

These exercises also help prevent contractures from developing in the limbs affected by stroke. A contracture is a shortening or shrinkage of muscle, tendon, ligament, or joint capsule that is caused by nonuse or infrequent use. It reduces a joint's range of motion and causes less overall mobility. Unless your doctor advises otherwise, do range-of-motion and stretching exercises using both the normal side of your body and the affected side. (The same applies to muscle-strengthening exercises.) This is important because stroke patients tend to underuse the limbs left weakened by stroke.[2]

At the beginning of an exercise session, and at the end if you have time (and I encourage you to make time), do several of the range-of-motion exercises and stretches shown and described in Figures 3.1-3.12 and 3.13-3.17. Over the years, I have found these to be particularly useful—provided exercisers follow these precautions:

- Check with your health-care team before performing any exercises that use one part of your body to foster a range-of-motion movement or stretch in another part of your body. For example,

Figure 3.13 shows an exercise where you use your left arm to stretch your right shoulder. Figures 3.14 and 3.16 also illustrate exercises of this type. For some stroke patients, such exercises are associated with a greater risk for injury.

- Do not stretch or do any of these exercises to the point where it becomes painful.
- Avoid sudden jerky movements, especially head movements. Abrupt changes in head position can precipitate strokes in susceptible people.[3]
- When doing exercises that involve turning your head to one side as far as possible, don't hold such a position for more than a few seconds. On at least one occasion, doctors found that such a head rotation, held for a couple of minutes, was a factor in triggering a stroke.[4]

Range-of-Motion Exercises

For all of the 12 range-of-motion exercises shown here, I recommend doing 3 to 5 repetitions of each. Bear in mind that joint range-of-motion exercises are meant to be done slowly with controlled movements. Also, you must discuss these exercises with your doctor before performing them to make sure they don't conflict with any residual neurological impairment you may still have.

Figure 3.1
Head Turns to Foster Neck Range of Motion. Look straight ahead. Keeping your eyes focused in the same plane, turn your head and look as far over your shoulder as possible. Hold that position for 2-3 seconds—but definitely no longer—and then return to your starting position. Repeat the same movement, looking over the other shoulder this time.

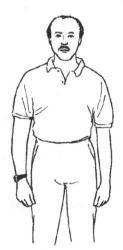
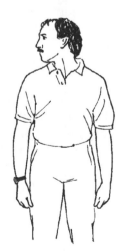

Figure 3.2
Head Tilt for Neck
Range of Motion. Keep
looking straight ahead as
you tilt your head so
that your left ear moves
toward your left shoul-
der. Hold that position
for 2-3 seconds, and
then return to your starting position. Repeat the
same movement with
the right ear and
shoulder.

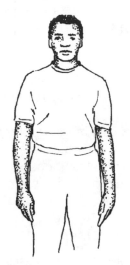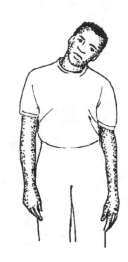

Figure 3.3
Arm Side-Raises for
Shoulder Range of Mo-
tion.   Stand with your
arms hanging at your
sides and your palms
against the outside of
your thighs. Raise both
arms sideways and up to-
ward your ears, while
allowing your elbows to
bend only slightly. Hold
that position for 2-3 seconds. Lower your arms
to the starting position
and repeat.

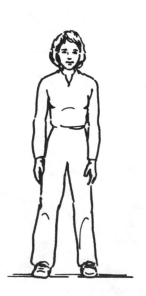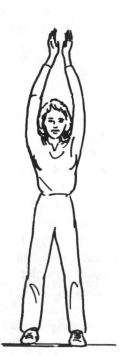

Figure 3.4
Shoulder Front-to-Back
Raises for Shoulder
Range of Motion.
Stand with your arms
hanging at your sides
and your palms facing
backwards. Raise your
one arm up in front of
you towards the ceiling,
all the while keeping
your elbow as straight as
possible. Simulta-
neously, raise your other
arm up behind you to-

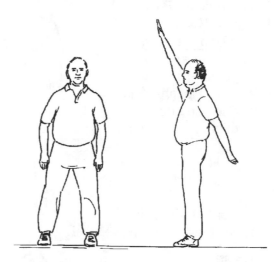

wards the ceiling, likewise keeping your elbow as straight as possible.
Hold that position for 2-3 seconds. Lower your arms to the starting
position and repeat, alternating the arms you move forward and back.

Figure 3.5
Shoulder-Blade Pulls for
Shoulder-Blade Range
of Motion.   Bend both elbows to a 90° angle. Lift
both elbows straight in
front of you and hold
them at shoulder level,
your palms facing down
and your upper arms
parallel to the floor. This
is your starting position.
Keeping your elbows
bent, pull them sideways

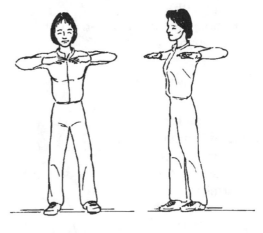

and backwards, whiletrying to pinch your shoulder blades together—a
position you should hold for 2-3 seconds. Return both elbows to the
starting position and repeat.

Figure 3.6
Side Bends for Back Range of Motion. Stand with your arms hanging at your sides and your palms against the outside of your thighs. Slide your one hand down your thigh, keeping your neck and back in a straight line and without leaning forward. Hold this position for 2-3 seconds. Return to the starting position and repeat with the other hand.

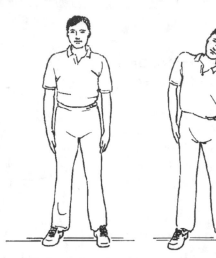

Figure 3.7
Elbow Curls for Elbow Range of Motion. Start with your arms hanging at your sides and your palms facing in front of you. Keeping your elbows close to your sides, curl both hands up toward your shoulders by bending your elbows. Hold this position for 2-3 seconds, then lower your hands to the starting position. Repeat

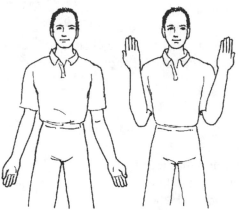

Figure 3.8
Wrist Circles for Wrist Range of Motion. Start with your arms hanging at your sides. While your arms remain stationary, move your hands in a circle in one direction and then in the other. Repeat.

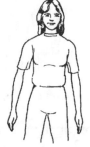
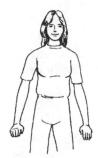

Figure 3.9
Finger Curls for Finger
Range of Motion. Start
with your arms hanging
at your sides and your
palms facing backward.
Curl all the fingers of
both hands—including
your thumbs—into a
loose fist. As you

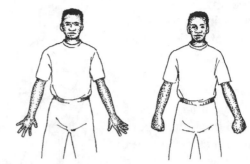

straighten your fingers, spread them as far apart
as possible. Repeat.

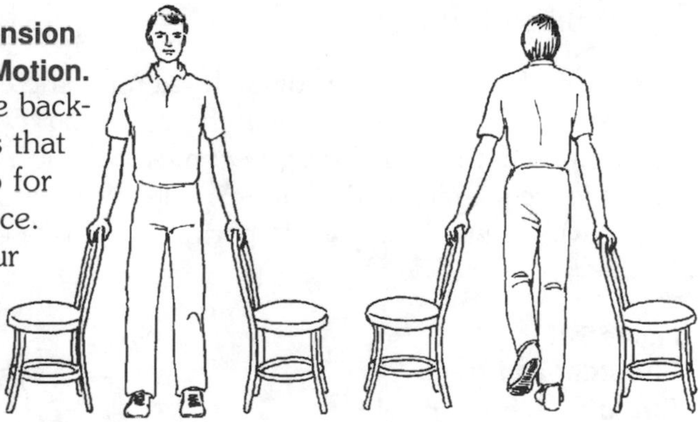

Figure 3.10
Standing Hip Extension
for Hip Range of Motion.
Stand between the back-
rests of two chairs that
you can hold onto for
support and balance.
While keeping your
back as straight
as possible, with
both knees
slightly bent and
one foot in place, press the other leg as far backward as possible and
lift it off the ground. Hold for 2-3 seconds. Return the leg to the
starting position and repeat with the other leg.

Figure 3.11
Supine Hip Abduction for
Hip Range of Motion. Lie
flat on your back with your
legs extended on the floor. Keeping
one leg straight in front of you,
slide the other leg as far out to
the side as possible. Hold
for 2-3 seconds. Return the
leg to the starting position and
repeat the same action with
the other leg.

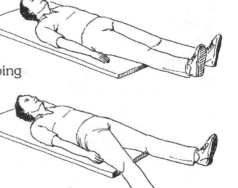

Figure 3.12
**Ankle Circles for Ankle
Range of Motion.** Sit
on the floor or on a
chair and extend one leg
out in front of you.
While your leg remains
stationary, move your
foot in a circle in one direction and then in the
other. Repeat with the
other foot.

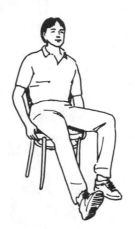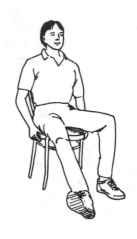

Stretching Exercises

Perform 1 to 3 repetitions of each exercise shown here. Hold each
stretch for 10 to 20 seconds with no bouncing. Don't ever stretch to
the point where the exercise becomes painful. Remember to keep
breathing regularly throughout—do not hold your breath. Once again,
check with your doctor before performing these exercises.

Figure 3.13
**Shoulder and Back
Stretch.** Lift your right
elbow toward the ceiling
and place your right
hand as far down your
back as possible between
the shoulder blades.
Allow your chin to rest
on your chest. If pos-
sible, using your left
hand, gently pull your
right elbow to the left until a stretch is felt on the
back of the right arm

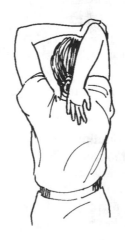

and down the right side of the back. Hold. Repeat with
the left arm.

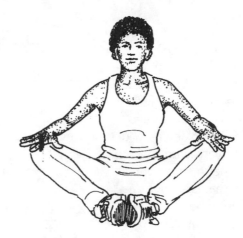

Figure 3.14
Inner Thigh Stretch. Sit on the floor, place the soles of your feet together, and pull your heels in as close to the buttocks as possible. Gently press your knees down toward the floor.

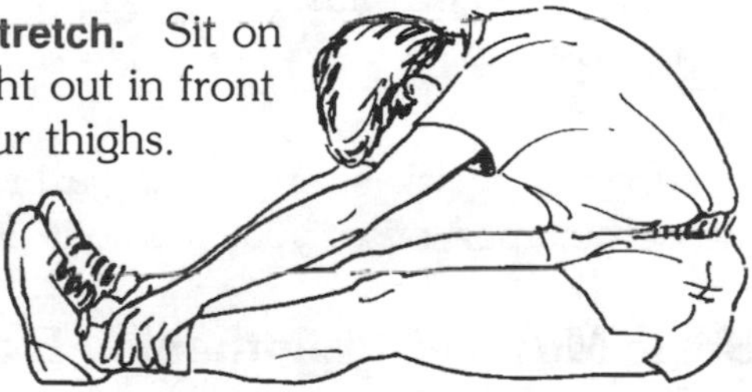

Figure 3.15
Lower Back and Hamstring Stretch. Sit on the floor with your legs straight out in front of you and your hands on your thighs. Bend forward slowly, reaching toward your toes. Keep your head and back aligned as you move into the stretch. If necessary, you can bend your knees slightly.

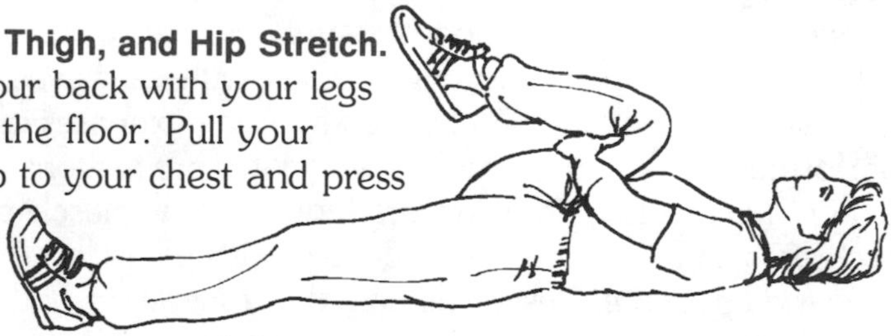

Figure 3.16
Lower Back, Thigh, and Hip Stretch. Lie flat on your back with your legs extended on the floor. Pull your right knee up to your chest and press your back to the floor. Hold this position and then repeat with the left knee.

Muscle-Strengthening Exercises

In contrast to flexibility training (which you should include in all your workouts), muscle-strengthening exercises need to be done only 2 or 3 days a week—and *not* on consecutive days. Also, if you prefer, you

Figure 3.17
Calf Stretch. Stand facing a wall, approximately 3 feet away. Place your palms on the wall, keeping your feet flat on the floor. Leave one foot in place as you step forward with the other. Make sure your back remains straight as you gently bend the front knee forward toward the wall. Repeat the same exercise with the opposite leg.

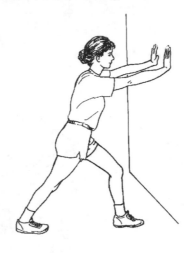

can do your muscle-strengthening exercises after, rather than before, the aerobic portion of your workout. It's up to you.

Basic Muscle-Strengthening Exercise Guidelines

Traditionally, doctors discouraged people with cardiovascular diseases (such as high blood pressure, heart conditions, or stroke) from doing muscle-strengthening exercises. Doctors feared these exercises could trigger a life-threatening cardiovascular event, because the exercises cause a marked rise in blood pressure.[5] Studies of stroke-prone rats with high blood pressure and humans with cardiovascular disease, however, suggest that muscle-strengthening exercises can, in fact, be performed safely, provided appropriate precautions are taken.[6-8] Other studies of stroke survivors indicate that muscle-strengthening programs can result in substantial strength gains, *even in the limbs affected by stroke.* Yes, be assured that muscle strengthening—done steadily and correctly over a reasonable period of time—is likely to increase your self-sufficiency and improve your ability to perform daily living activities.[9]

If your doctor clears you to proceed with strengthening exercises, pay special attention to the following words of caution:

- *Never hold a contraction for more than about 6 seconds because this could cause an excessive rise in your blood pressure.* Isometric exercise—a static type of muscle strengthening in which a muscle remains contracted for more than a few seconds without relaxing—can elicit adverse cardiac responses in stroke patients.

• *Avoid holding your breath because it places increased stress on your cardiovascular system.* A Valsalva maneuver during lifting—that is, exhaling forcefully without releasing the air from the lungs—is ill-advised. Breathe out (exhale) on the most strenuous part of an exercise.

• *Do not undertake activities where you must hold weight above your head for more than a few seconds.* Such movements also place an excessive load on your cardiovascular system.

• *Substitute lighter weights for heavier weights and do more repetitions.* Do not use heavier weights, or greater resistance, with the idea that you'll exercise for a shorter time. Heavier weights increase your blood pressure more than lighter ones.

• *Don't strain!* You should not exceed a Borg RPE of 13 during muscular conditioning (see the Borg Perceived Exertion Scale on page 48).

Muscle-Strengthening Exercises Using Resistance Rubber Bands

I've developed an easy muscle-strengthening program you can do at home that is based on the use of special rubber bands. Many people who have had strokes and many elderly people prefer these bands to hand-held weights because they're easier to grip. The bands are inexpensive, versatile, and convenient to use, and several types are available. (Dyna-Bands and Therabands, two of the most popular, can be ordered from The Hygenic Corporation, 1245 Home Ave., Akron, OH 44310; phone, 216-633-8460.)

Here's how to exercise with these bands. Either pull or push against the bands, which resist your efforts. The amount of resistance varies according to the thickness of the band, and the bands are color-coded to indicate thickness. If necessary, use a thinner, less resistant band when exercising the side of your body affected by stroke. You can exercise with one band only or use them in combination for greater resistance.

Here are some more exercise safety tips to bear in mind:

• Before you begin to exercise, remove all jewelry from your arms, even your watch.
• For some of the exercises, you'll need to tie your band so it forms a loop. Use a knot or a half-bow, which is easier to undo.
• During an exercise, always try to maintain the natural width of the band. Don't let it fold over.

- Maintain good posture throughout the exercise sequence.
- Start slowly and progress gradually. If you're weak to start with, it won't take much exercise to improve your strength. In fact, one study found that people with weak muscles can increase their strength dramatically just by performing their exercise program working against gravity, without adding any resistance or weight at all.[10] When using the bands, start with the thinner ones and progress to thicker ones only if you can tolerate them.

My program works all the major muscles and was designed specifically for stroke patients and people with other chronic diseases. You can do these exercises at home with little risk of adverse consequences. Still, you should check with your doctor before starting. The program is depicted in Figures 3.18-3.28.

I recommend that you do these exercises 3 days a week on alternate days, following these guidelines:

- If you find it difficult to hold the band in your hand without it slipping out, you may need to tie loops at each end and attach them around your hands or wrists. If you do this, you'll need to order bands longer than the standard 36 inches (91 cm). Another option is to buy special handles.
- When wrapping a band around any part of your body, do it so you're still comfortable. It should never be too tight.
- Begin your exercise sequence with the thinnest band, which provides the least resistance. As tolerance permits, gradually progress to the thicker bands.
- For each exercise, do 12-20 slow, complete, and controlled repetitions. Each execution should take 3-5 seconds, and your movements should be smooth and continuous. Never jerk your band or allow it to snap back. Always keep some tension on the band as it returns to its starting position; you can relax completely for 2-3 seconds between repetitions. You control the band. Don't let it control you.
- Rest for 15-60 seconds between each set. (The full number of repetitions ordered for each exercise is referred to as a *set*.) Once you've reached the point where, with relative ease, you can do two complete sets (2 × 20 repetitions for each exercise), you may want to progress to a thicker, more resistant band. However, keep in mind that it's far more important to do the exercises correctly than to increase the amount of resistance.

Figure 3.18
Side Shoulder Raise
(outer portion of the
shoulders). Place your
foot on one end of the
band and grip the other
end with the hand on
the opposite side of your
body. Start with your
arm extended at your
side and the palm of
your hand facing the
side of your thigh. Keep-
ing your elbow slightly
bent, raise your arm out

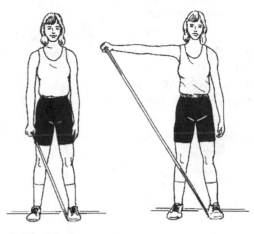

at your side to shoulder level. Slowly lower
your arm to the starting position. Repeat this
motion with the same arm until you fulfill your repetition goal.
Then switch to the other arm and leg and repeat.

Figure 3.19
Front Shoulder Raise
(front portion of the
shoulders). This is a
variation of Figure 3.18.
Once again, place your
foot on one end of the
band, but this time grip
the other end with the
hand on the same side
of your body. Begin with
your arm extended at
your side and the palm
of your hand facing the
side of your thigh. Raise
your arm out in front of
your body to shoulder

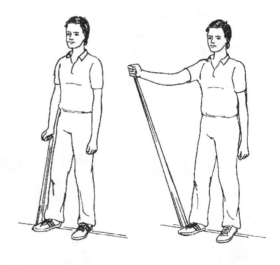

level. Slowly lower your arm to the starting position. Repeat this
motion with the same arm until you fulfill your repetition goal.
Then switch to the other arm and leg and repeat.

**Figure 3.20
Chest Press (chest muscles and upper back).**
Loop the band around your upper back and grip the ends in your hands. Bend both elbows to a 90° angle. Lift both elbows away from your sides until they're at armpit level and your arms are almost parallel to the floor. This is your starting position. Press your arms forward until they're almost completely straight. Slowly bend your elbows until your hands return to the starting position. Repeat.

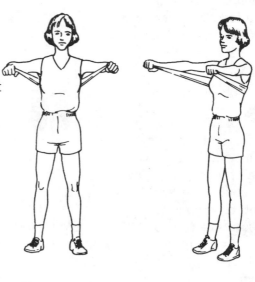

**Figure 3.21
Biceps Curl (muscles in the front of the upper arm).** Place your foot on one end of the band and grip the other end with the hand on the same side of your body. Start with your arm extended at your side and the palm of your hand facing forward. Keeping your elbow close to your side, bend it so that your fist curls upward to your shoulder. Slowly lower your arm to the starting

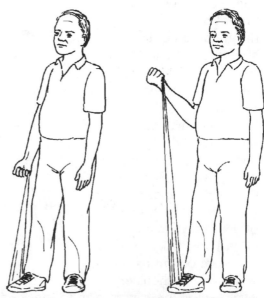

position. Repeat this motion with the same armuntil you fulfill your repetition goal. Then switch to the other arm and leg and repeat.

Figure 3.22
Triceps Extension (muscles in the back of the upper arm). Take one step forward and place your front foot on one end of the band. Grip the other end with the hand on the opposite side of your body. Bend your front knee slightly, lean forward, and rest the hand on the same side of the body, palm down, on your knee. Place the other hand—the one holding the band—against your hip, palm facing inward. Gradually straighten that arm out fully behind you. Then slowly bend your arm until your hand returns to the starting position at your hip. Repeat this motion with the same arm until you fulfill your repetition goal. Then switch to the opposite arm and leg and repeat.

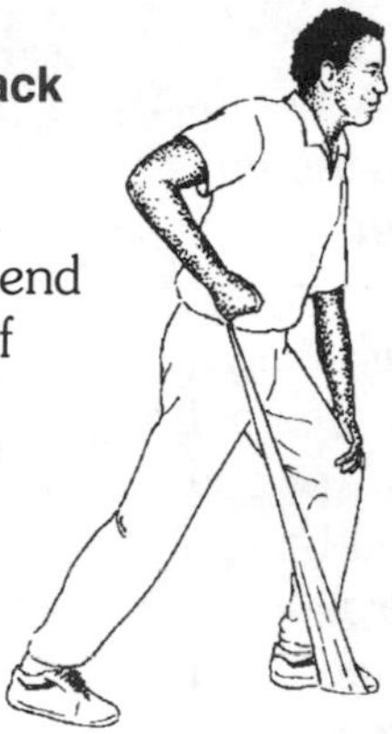

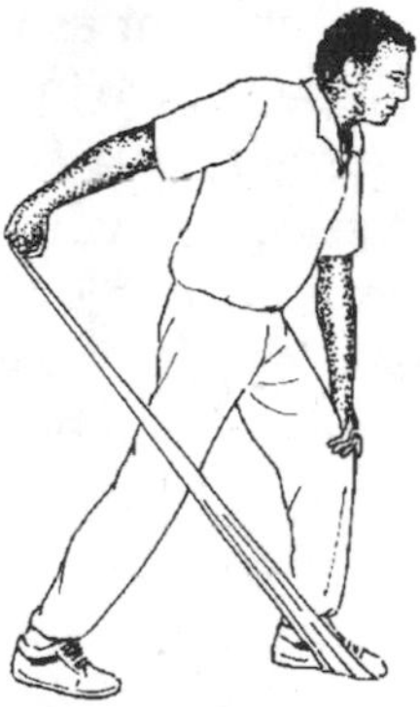

Figure 3.23
Seated Rowing Exercise (upper back, shoulders, and neck). Sit on the floor with your back upright and your knees either bent or straight, whichever is more comfortable. Grab each end of the band with your hands and loop the band around your feet. Start with your arms extended in front of you, your hands slightly lower than shoulder level, and your palms facing the floor. Pull both ends of the band toward your armpits, while maintaining good posture. Slowly return your hands to the starting position and repeat.

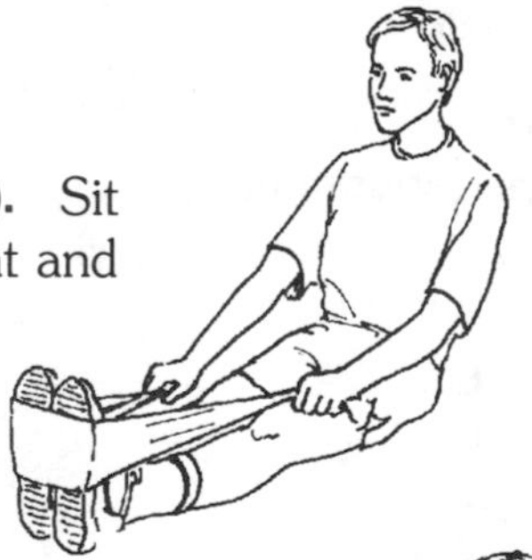

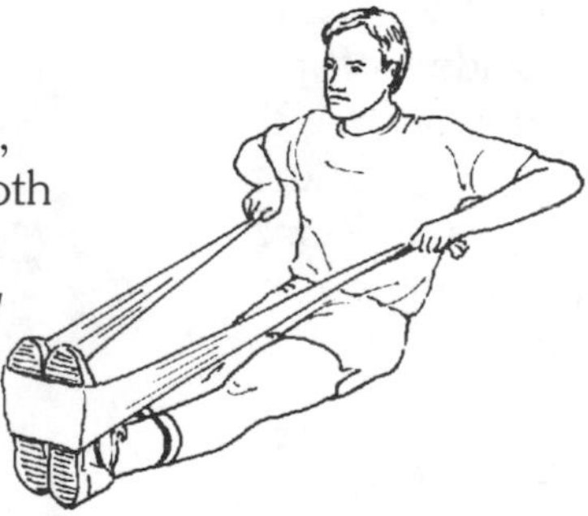

Figure 3.24
Seated Hip Abduction
(hips and outer
thighs).   Sit on the
floor with your back up-
right and your legs out
straight in front of you.
Place a knotted band
around the outside of
your ankles. Keep your
legs straight as you
brace yourself with
palms on the floor

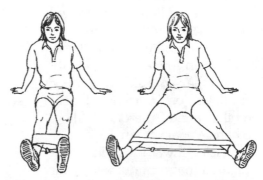

just behind you. Slide your legs apart until you note significant
resistance. Slowly return both legs to the starting position
and repeat. To decrease the resistance, do this exercise with the
band looped around the outside of your thighs just above the
knees.

Figure 3.25
Half-Sit-Ups (abdominal
muscles).   Lie on the
floor with your knees
bent at a 90° angle and
the palms of your hands
resting on the front of
your thighs. Lift your
shoulders off the floor
and slide your fingers up
toward your knees. Re-
turn to the horizontal
starting position and re-
peat.

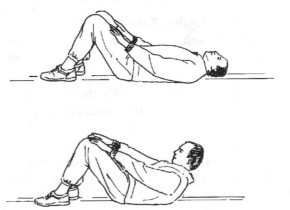

Figure 3.26
Standing Hip Flexion (hips and the front of the thighs). Stand between the backrests of two chairs with your feet close together. Place a looped band around the outside of your ankles. Throughout this exercise, hold onto both backrests for balance and support and keep both knees slightly bent. Bracing yourself with your arms and keeping one foot in place, press the other leg forward until you encounter significant resistance. Slowly return your leg to the starting position and repeat with the opposite leg. For less resistance, do this exercise with the looped band around the outside of your thighs just above the knees.

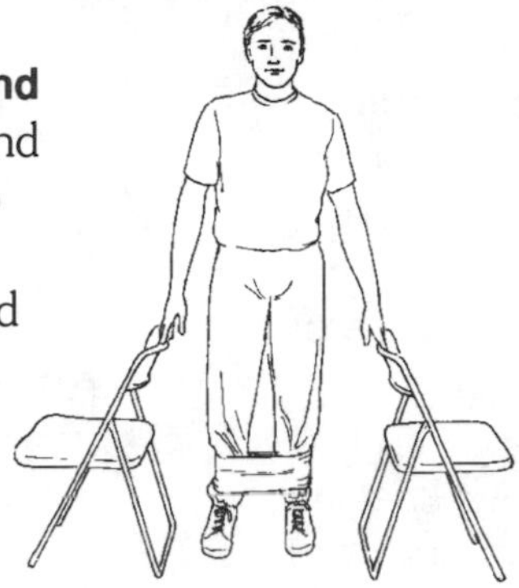

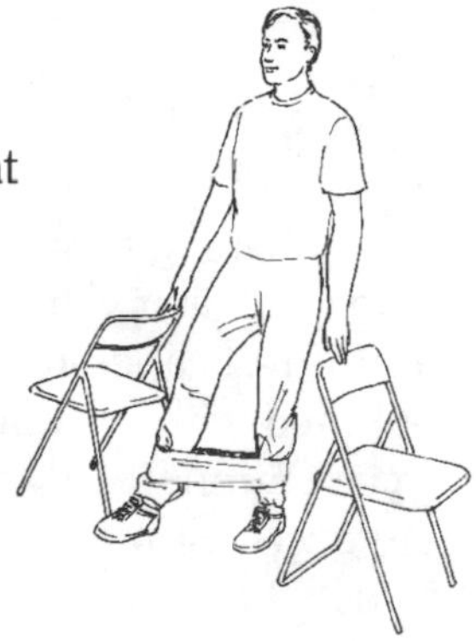

Figure 3.27
Standing Hip Extension (hips, back of the thighs, buttocks, and lower back muscles). Stand between the backrests of two chairs with your feet close together. Place a looped band around the outside of your ankles. Throughout this exercise hold onto both backrests for balance and support and keep both knees slightly bent. Bracing yourself with your arms and keeping one foot in place, press the other leg backward until you encounter significant resistance. Slowly return your leg to the starting position and repeat with the opposite leg. For less resistance, do this exercise with the looped band around the outside of your thighs just above the knees.

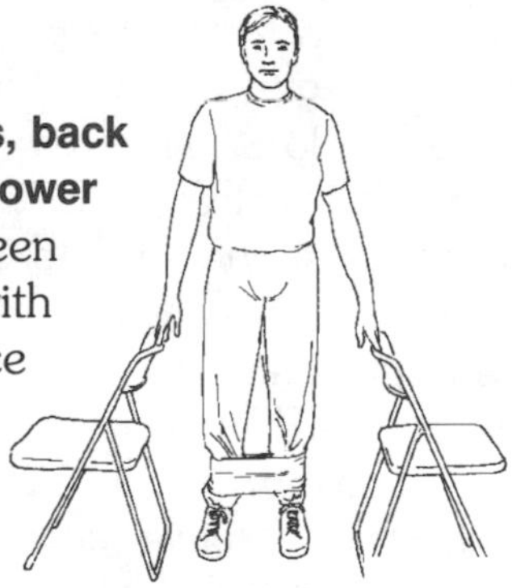

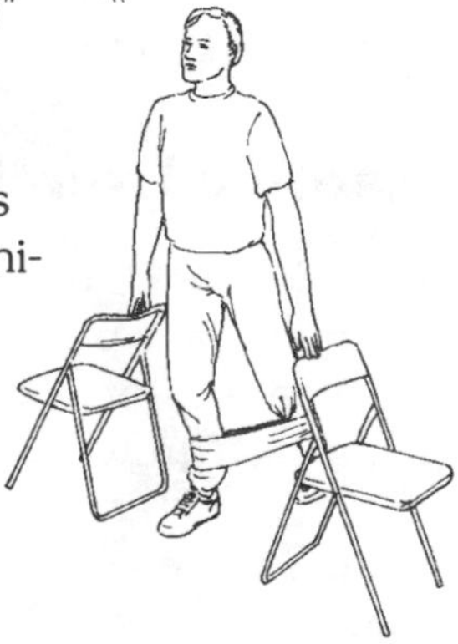

Figure 3.28
Calf Raises (calf muscles).   Stand with your hands against a wall in front of you for balance. Rise up onto the balls of both feet. Lower your heels to the floor and repeat. Keep your knees straight throughout this exercise.

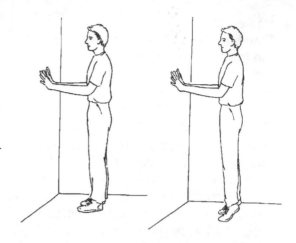

If your doctor clears you to undertake a more strenuous muscle-strengthening program, find an adequately trained health professional who is familiar with your case and willing to instruct you in the correct use of resistance-training equipment. A well-equipped gym might be outfitted with weight-training devices carrying such brand names as Cybex Strength Systems, Hydrafitness, Nautilus, and Universal. These are excellent machines, but someone should carefully teach you how to use them and supervise your exercise.

The American College of Sports Medicine recommends that the average healthy adult do a minimum of 8 to 10 exercises involving the major muscle groups at least twice weekly. They further encourage adults to perform at least one set (8 to 12 repetitions) of each muscle-strengthening exercise during each of these workouts.[11] These recommendations are appropriate for people who have had a stroke, with one notable exception. I encourage stroke patients instead to *use lighter weights* and *do more consecutive repetitions* of an exercise— between 12 and 20 consecutive repetitions for each exercise.[12] Such an approach lessens the rise in blood pressure during exercise.

Aerobic Exercise

Ken Cooper coined the term *aerobics* in 1968, when his first book, *Aerobics*, was published.[13] If you'd looked up the word *aerobic* in the dictionary before 1968, it would have been described as an adjective meaning "growing in air or in oxygen." It was commonly used to describe bacteria that need oxygen to live. Ken, however, used the word *aerobics* as a noun to denote those forms of endurance exercises that require increased amounts of oxygen for prolonged periods of time. Proof of Ken's influence came in the 1986 edition of the *Oxford English Dictionary*, in which *aerobics* is defined as "a method of physical exercise for producing beneficial changes in the respiratory and circulatory systems by activities which require only a modest increase of oxygen intake and so can be maintained."

How much aerobic exercise is just enough to insure health benefits without increasing the chances of injury or medical emergency? Steven N. Blair, director of epidemiology at The Cooper Institute for Aerobics Research, and researchers from other medical institutions (including the Centers for Disease Control, Stanford University, and the University of Wisconsin) have examined this issue in depth.[14-16] They reviewed the findings of many exercise research studies and identified an ideal upper and lower limit of exercise. In other words (although future studies are needed to clarify the situation), there does appear to be a just-right level of exercise. That level is a modest amount, far less than the extremely strenuous workouts that exercise enthusiasts engage in as a matter of course. In the language of exercise physiologists,

> Exercise training that results in a weekly energy expenditure of between *10 and 20 calories per kilogram of body weight** is likely to bring about major health benefits.[14, 15] Twenty calories is the upper limit necessary from a health promotion standpoint—energy expenditures above this level do not appear to provide substantially more benefit.[14] The lower limit of 10 calories is necessary to insure effectiveness,[15] although lesser amounts are still likely to be of some benefit.[17]

Here are two examples: Roger weighed 196 pounds (89 kilograms) when he first arrived at The Cooper Aerobics Center. He needed to gradually build up to an energy expenditure of between 890 (89 × 10) and 1,780 (89 × 20) calories during exercise each week. Another stroke patient, Lynne, weighed 132 pounds (60 kilograms). Her target weekly energy expenditure during exercise was 600 (60 × 10) to 1,200 (60 × 20) calories.

The conclusions just described form the mathematical basis of the Health Points System described in the next chapter. Most patients would find it difficult to figure out how much exercise they need to do to expend 10 to 20 calories per kilogram of body weight. Fortunately, our Health Points System transforms these seemingly complicated energy expenditure recommendations into a practical,

---

*1 kilogram (kg) = approximately 2.2 pounds. 1 calorie = approximately 4.2 kilojoules.

easy-to-follow method to assess your exercise program. So if you're concerned about the complexity of calculating your weekly energy expenditure, you can stop worrying. Our Health Points System will take care of this for you.

Factors That Determine Energy Expenditure

Weekly energy expenditure during exercise depends largely on four factors: the *type, frequency, intensity*, and *duration* of your exercise sessions. It's your health-care team's job to use these four elements to help tailor a safe and effective weekly exercise program for you. Keeping both your medical condition and personal preferences in mind, your health-care team must help you do the following:

- Choose a suitable aerobic exercise.
- Decide on the number of times you should work out each week.
- Determine the appropriate exercise intensity.
- Establish how long each session should last.

It's important for you to understand how the last three items intertwine. They're embodied in the concept of FIT, which is an acronym for **F**requency, **I**ntensity, and **T**ime. If you exercise regularly, you're undoubtedly familiar with this notion already. *Frequency* refers to *how often* you exercise. *Intensity* refers to *how hard* you exert yourself. *Time* refers to each exercise session's *duration*. An equation showing their interrelationship would look like this:

$$\textbf{F}\text{requency} + \textbf{I}\text{ntensity} + \textbf{T}\text{ime} = \text{Caloric energy expenditure}$$
$$= \text{Health benefit}$$

Clearly, if the amount on the right side of the equation (caloric energy expenditure and health benefit) remains constant and you cut down on one or two elements on the left side of the equation, the third element on the left side of the equation must increase to make up the difference. For example, if you exercise at a low to moderate intensity 3 days a week, each exercise session may have to last a relatively long time if you're to get enough exercise to have a substantial impact on your health. On the other hand, you may choose instead to exercise at the same low to moderate intensity but for a shorter length of time each session. In this instance, you'll have to increase the number of times per week that you exercise to achieve the desired weekly energy expenditure.

Here are my recommendations concerning each of these factors:

Frequency.   For healthy people, I recommend 3 to 5 days per week as the ideal exercise schedule. And my advice is the same for stroke survivors. Fewer is unlikely to produce significant health improvements; more predisposes you to musculoskeletal injuries. And space your workouts throughout the week. For example, if you're a 3-day-a-week exerciser, rather than training on Monday, Tuesday, and Wednesday, you'd be better off exercising on Monday, Wednesday, and Friday.

Time or Duration.   As I discussed, the higher the intensity or frequency, the shorter the time needed to attain the desired weekly energy expenditure. Moderate-intensity aerobic exercise of longer duration is preferable to high-intensity exercise of shorter duration for stroke patients for these reasons: (a) It lessens the risk of training-related medical complications. (b) It is less stressful on your musculoskeletal system. (c) The average person is more likely to enjoy more moderate workouts. (d) Many patients simply cannot exercise at high intensities because of partial paralysis and other neurological impairments caused by stroke. Longer, moderate workouts are particularly important if weight loss is a goal because they promote fat loss while reducing the risk of musculoskeletal injuries.[12]

For most of you, workouts of 30 to 45 minutes of continuous aerobic exercise are the goal you should aim to gradually build up to. But preliminary research at Stanford University offers an alternative. It shows that three 10-minute exercise sessions spread throughout the day may result in fitness gains similar to one 30-minute session.[18] This finding should be welcome news to those of you who prefer shorter exercise sessions.

Remember, these recommendations on duration do not include the warm-up and cool-down periods, which should open and close each aerobics session. Take at least 5 minutes to ease into aerobics, starting at a low intensity and slowly building up to your peak, target intensity. You should also reduce your exercise intensity gradually for 5 minutes at the end of your workout.

Intensity.   The notion that you must exercise at high intensities to obtain health benefits is a fallacy. In short, the "no pain, no gain" axiom is wrong. It's also an especially dangerous idea for anyone who is prone to hemorrhagic strokes or who has such other chronic diseases as hypertension, heart disease, diabetes, or arthritis. Fortunately, you can obtain optimal health benefits with a minimum of risk by exercising at moderate rather than high intensity.

How to Quantify Exercise Intensity

There are a number of ways to quantify exercise intensity, and I'll discuss three: metabolic equivalent units (METs), heart rate, and perceived exertion.

METs.   One MET is the amount of oxygen your body consumes for energy production each minute while you're at rest. If you're engaged in an activity corresponding to 5 METs, this means that your body is taking up and using five times more oxygen than it did at rest. This is the amount it now needs to fuel your working muscles, enabling them to produce the required amount of energy. (I'll discuss METs later in this chapter when I explain how to select an appropriate speed or work rate for the initial weeks of a walking or stationary cycling exercise program.)

Heart Rate.   This is perhaps the most widely used and helpful way to target exercise intensity. It's based on the principle that there's a direct relationship between the increase in your body's oxygen uptake during exertion and the increase in your heart rate.

I advise my stroke patients to exercise at an intensity that raises the heart rate above 60% of their maximal heart rate but no higher than 85%; that's an exercise training zone range spanning 25 percentage points. I have found that an exercise heart rate in the range of 60% to 75% of the maximal heart rate is ideal for most stroke patients, especially those with high blood pressure.[7]

What's your maximal heart rate? The figure varies between individuals. Your maximal heart rate is the highest heart rate that you can attain during exercise without developing any significant cardiovascular abnormalities.

The most accurate way to determine your maximal heart rate is to have a treadmill test or, alternatively, a cycle test that makes you work either your legs or your arms, or both. At the Cooper Clinic, we insist that all our stroke survivors take an exercise test before they begin a regular exercise program. Not only that, we encourage our stroke patients to take a follow-up test if they change certain medications, develop a new medical problem, or experience a significant change in an existing medical condition, either for better or worse.

In medical jargon, this test is called a "symptom-limited maximal exercise test with electrocardiogram (ECG) and blood pressure monitoring." The term *symptom-limited* simply means that you exercise until you cannot continue because either you are too fatigued or you develop certain ECG, blood pressure, or other abnormalities that indicate to your physician that the test should be stopped. Why is the test so crucial? Because it enables your doctor to tell you the highest heart rate you can achieve without developing any cardiovascular abnormalities. *This is the value you should use as your maximal heart rate.*

Both Roger and Lynne had exercise tests. Roger's maximal heart rate was 145 beats per minute. Lynne's was 140 beats per minute. If you don't have a test, you can use the following formula to *estimate* your maximal heart rate:

> 220 minus your age in years = Estimated maximal heart rate

For example, Roger at age 68 had an estimated maximal heart rate of 152 beats per minute (220 − 68 = 152). At age 71, Lynne's estimated maximal heart rate was 149 beats per minute (220 − 71 = 149) before she began our supervised exercise program. Note that Roger's actual maximal heart rate (145) was slightly lower than his estimate. Lynne's (140) was also lower.

This formula is invalid for people taking medications (such as beta blockers) that slow the heart rate. For safety reasons, I also caution people who know or suspect they have heart disease to ignore this formula—whether or not they're taking medication. People in this category must have an exercise test.

Training Target Heart Rate Zone. Once you know your maximal heart rate—either estimated using the formula or based on an exercise test—it's easy to determine the heart rate levels you should stay within when you exercise. As I mentioned previously, I recommend that you exercise at an intensity above 60% of your maximal heart rate but no higher than 75% (and definitely not above 85%). This is your *training target heart rate zone.* You can calculate it by multiplying your maximal heart rate by the lower limit of 60% (or 0.6) and by the upper limit of 75% (or 0.75).

Using Roger's actual maximal heart rate of 145, he calculated a lower limit of 87 beats per minute (145 × 0.6 = 87) and an upper limit of 109 beats per minute (145 × 0.75 = 109). Lynne's training target heart rate zone was between 84 (140 × 0.6 = 84) and 105 (140 × 0.75 = 105) beats per minute.

This zone is important. Studies show that exercising at an intensity lower than 60% may net you some health benefits but is unlikely to substantially increase your fitness level. Also, if you don't exceed the 60% mark, you'll probably have to lengthen each exercise session to well over an hour to attain the recommended weekly energy expenditure. But if you are under time pressure and can work out only 3 days a week or for short durations, you'll need to exercise near the upper limit of your training target heart rate zone to gain appreciable health benefits.

Some stroke patients are so physically unfit that they become quickly fatigued at intensities that raise their heart rate above 60%. For these patients interval training is better than one long, endurance-oriented workout. They should exercise in a series of bouts at the desired intensity, each separated by a short rest period, or period of very low-intensity exertion.

Remember, it's crucial to never exceed the 85% upper limit. Why? Because high-intensity exercise increases the risk for triggering cardiovascular complications during exercise.

Using Heart Rate to Guide Intensity.   For those new to exercise, the questions and answers that follow offer insight into how to use heart rate as a guide to exercise intensity:

• *How do I measure my heart rate during exercise?* The same way you'd do it at rest—by taking your pulse. (See Appendix A.)

• *How often during exercise should I calculate my heart rate?* Initially, you may need to check your heart rate as often as every 5 minutes. But after you are familiar with your appropriate exercise intensity, you may need to do it only a few times each workout. I generally recommend that you check your rate at the following times:

1. Before starting to exercise. If it is above 100 beats per minute and remains this high after 15 minutes or so of rest, don't exercise at all. Check with your doctor to see why it's so high.
2. After you complete your warm-up. If your heart rate is above your upper heart rate limit at this point, slow down until it drops below the upper limit. You performed your warm-up at too high an intensity. Start off slower next time.
3. After you've been exercising at your peak intensity for about 5 minutes. If it is above your upper limit, slow down and recheck it in 5 minutes.
4. When you stop the aerobic phase and begin your cool-down.
5. When you complete your cool-down. If your heart rate isn't below 100 beats per minute, rest until it reaches this level. Only then should you take a shower or drive off in your car.

• *Can I rely on a portable heart rate monitor instead of checking my heart rate manually?* Commercially available meters are generally worn on the chest and provide continual monitoring of your heart rate by transmitting electrical signals to a special wristwatch or to a computer that's also worn on your chest. Usually, you can program your heart rate limit into the device, and it will set off an alarm if you exceed it. Provided you purchase a reliable model, such monitors can be helpful, but they're certainly not a necessity.

Consult a member of your health-care team before buying one. Ask which type he or she thinks is most accurate. Then before you buy a specific one, ask that team member to help you verify its accuracy while you're wearing it.

Defining Exercise Intensity by Perceived Exertion.   One of the simplest ways to measure your exercise intensity is to use the Borg scale reproduced in Table 3.1. Named after the Swedish exercise physiologist Gunnar Borg who developed it in the early 1950s, the Borg scale helps you judge your exercise intensity based on your on-the-spot

Table 3.1
Borg Perceived Exertion Scale

The original Borg system for rating physical exertion is based on an open-ended scale running from 6 (equal to exertion at rest) to 20 (extreme effort).

Rating of perceived exertion or RPE	Verbal description of RPE
6	
7	Very, very light
8	
9	Very light
10	
11	Fairly light
12	
13	Somewhat hard
14	
15	Hard
16	
17	Very hard
18	
19	Very, very hard
20	

Note. From G.A. Borg, "Psychophysical Bases of Perceived Exertion," *Medicine and Science in Sports and Exercise, 14*, pp. 377-387, 1982, © by The American College of Sports Medicine. Reprinted by permission.

perception of how hard the exercise feels.[19] This rating of perceived exertion (RPE) is outlined on a scale from 6 to 20, which you consult as you exercise. If you're exerting yourself at a level that you feel is fairly strenuous, you might assign your effort an RPE of 13. When you reach the all-out huffing-and-puffing stage, you'd choose a much higher rating of about 17.

Generally, an RPE of 12 to 13 corresponds to an exercise intensity of 60% to 75% of your maximal heart rate. In other words, the 12-to-13 RPE range corresponds to your training target heart rate zone, which you should aim for during the aerobic portion of your workout. Never exceed a score of 15, even if your heart rate is below your prescribed limit.

Basic Aerobic Exercises to Get You Started

Aerobic exercises *don't* require excessive speed or strength, but they *do* require that you place some demands on your cardiovascular system. In contrast, anaerobic means without oxygen. Sprinting is an anaerobic activity. It involves an all-out burst of effort and relies on metabolic processes that do not require oxygen for energy production. Such activities cause fatigue within a relatively short period of time.

Of the two types, aerobic exercise is far better for stroke patients who want to improve their health for these reasons: Energy expenditure is related to how much oxygen your working muscles use during exercise. Aerobic exercise obviously uses more oxygen than anaerobic exercise. Also, because it's more moderate and you can do it longer, aerobic exercise allows you to expend far more energy than anaerobic exercise. And when you exercise aerobically, you can better monitor your heart rate and keep it within your prescribed limit. Anaerobic exercise is more likely to push your heart rate above that limit, which can be dangerous if you have cardiovascular disease. Anaerobic exercise is also likely to cause an excessive rise in your blood pressure.

The beginning aerobic exercises I most commonly recommend for stroke patients with no or only slight-to-moderate disabilities are walking, cycling, and, for those with Grade 1 disability (see chapter 2), sometimes even jogging. Each has its pluses and minuses.

Walking.   Most stroke experts, including me, consider walking one of the most appropriate aerobic activities for those who can do it. According to one study, one year after a stroke, 32% of stroke survivors can walk just as well as they did before, and almost 50% can walk with no assistance or with a cane.[20]

Walking requires no equipment other than a good pair of shoes, and it's unlikely to cause or aggravate musculoskeletal problems. The intensity is easy to control, so even many stroke patients with other chronic diseases can walk and get the desired conditioning effect. And a recent study by Tom R. Thomas and Ben R. Londeree suggests that the energy expenditure for walking at fast speeds approaches that for jogging.[21]

For walking with a cane or other support aid on a level surface, here is the correct sequence of movements: (a) Hold the cane in your *unaffected* hand and advance the cane first. (b) Next, move your *affected* leg forward. (c) Step forward with your *unaffected* leg. The height of your cane should be such that there's a slight 15° bend in your elbow when you stand erect with your hand on the cane at your side. Never lean on the cane with a straight elbow; this will put undue strain on both your elbow and wrist.

For more information on walking after a stroke and for general information about stroke recovery, I highly recommend the National Stroke Association's excellent book, *The Road Ahead: A Stroke Recovery Guide.*[22]

Jogging. For stroke patients who can jog, the benefits are similar to those for walking. The catch is that when you jog, your feet strike the ground with a force that's usually equal to three to four times your body weight. This force is transmitted to your weight-bearing joints and, over time and done to excess, predisposes you to musculoskeletal injuries. In contrast to jogging, walking exerts a force of only 1 to 1-1/2 times your weight on the weight-bearing joints.[23] Also, jogging generally requires greater exertion, or intensity, than walking, thus often inducing a heart rate higher than your limit. But if you're enthusiastic about jogging despite the greater risks that may accompany it (and if you are capable of doing it), I recommend that your jogging program be preceded by a walking program, then a walk/jog regimen. When approached in a sensible manner, many patients with no residual neurological impairments can eventually include jogging in their training program with success.

Stationary Cycling. Busy people love this activity. While you're pedaling away on your stationary cycle (also known as a *cycle ergometer*), you can do other things—read or watch TV, for example. Stationary cycling gives you no excuse should the weather make outdoor cycling impossible, and it causes less wear and tear on the musculoskeletal system than many aerobic activities, including even walking. To reduce the stress on your knees, set the saddle height so that your knee joints straighten almost fully during pedaling.

Stationary cycling has a few disadvantages, though. Some people who've had a stroke aren't stable enough to sit on a stationary bike. If you're one of them, you may have to skip this exercise. Another drawback is that during a long ride, you may develop sore buttocks. If you have no loss of sensation as a result of your stroke, you'll recognize this discomfort, which occurs from being in one position too long. It can be remedied simply by shifting your buttocks every now and then. If you have lost buttocks sensation, you'll have to remember to shift every few minutes to prevent pressure sores. Because of such problems, I often advise patients to combine stationary cycling with walking.

Some stationary cycles, such as the Schwinn Air-Dyne, work your arms and legs simultaneously, which helps you achieve higher energy expenditures. You pump your legs up and down while you move your arms forward and back. The result is a more thorough upper- and lower-body workout with less stress on your lower-limb joints. I recommend these machines for many of our stroke patients, especially those who use their arms a lot in their jobs or for recreation.

For those of you who can use the arm and leg on only one side of the body, or who are unstable sitting on a stationary bike, it's possible to alter the Schwinn Air-Dyne and some other bikes. I've seen patients who use a wheelchair use their good arm and leg to work specially modified bikes.[24]

Arm-Cycle Ergometry.   This is one alternative for patients who cannot use their legs during exercise but whose arms are relatively unaffected. The downside of arm-cycle ergometry is that because the upper-limb muscles are smaller than those of the lower limb, you have to work much harder to achieve a given energy expenditure. Also, for a given rise in heart rate, it causes a greater rise in blood pressure, especially if you can use only one of your arms.

If you use a wheelchair, an alternative to arm-cycle ergometry is to simply use your arms to propel yourself along in your chair. When correctly performed, wheelchair exercise can yield major health benefits.[25, 26] But make sure the terrain you're traversing is level and unencumbered. The last thing you need is to injure yourself. Wheelchair exercisers should also wear gloves to prevent blisters and have good seat cushioning to prevent pressure sores.

Outdoor Cycling.   In my opinion, outdoor cycling is far more enjoyable and exhilarating than pedaling away indoors. The disadvantage over a stationary workout is that roads tend to go up and down. So an outdoor cyclist needs more stability, balance, and coordination— qualities that stroke patients are often deficient in. Also, an unexpected incline could cause your heart rate to rise too high. And too many downhill stretches and delays at stoplights may lessen your energy expenditure so much that you need to exercise longer to meet the desired energy expenditure. Then, of course, there is the problem of riding in traffic—it's dangerous. Still, if you're sure you can handle these conditions, outdoor cycling is a great way to exercise.

PUTTING ON THOSE WALKING SHOES AND VENTURING FORTH

This section offers guidelines on initiating a walking, walk/jog, or stationary cycling exercise program. I recommend these forms of exercise to stroke patients because they're a good way to slowly ease into the routine of regular exercise.

After you've completed an introductory 10 to 12 weeks or so of one of the following programs, you'll be ready to start trying to earn the 50 to 100 exercise health points I discuss in the next chapter.

Please note that these programs are intended as guidelines. Your individual circumstances may require you to progress more slowly.

Beginning Walking Program

Walking is a wonderful way for many stroke patients to get moving down the road to optimal health. But before you begin, you should know your maximal MET value so you can estimate the speed (in mph or kph) at which you should walk during the first 12 weeks. Your maximal MET value depends on your fitness level and the neurological impairment caused by your stroke. If you've undergone an exercise test (which I urge all stroke patients to do), your doctor can provide you with your maximal MET value. If not, err on the side of caution. Start at a comfortable speed that does not exceed what's recommended in Table 3.2 on page 56 for a person with a maximal MET value of 5. Regardless of whether you know your maximal MET value, I strongly advise against exceeding 75% of your maximal heart rate and an RPE of 13 during the initial weeks. Table 3.2 shows what your estimated beginning walking speed should be. Using this table, Roger Knight, whose maximal MET value was 4, started his walking program at a speed of about 1.8 mph, or 2.9 kph.

The box on page 56 shows you what your walking program will look like in terms of each workout's duration and frequency.

A Follow-Up Walk-Jog Program

Don't try jogging until you've followed a walking regimen for at least 6 weeks, ideally 12 weeks. In your walking program, you should be walking at speeds in excess of 4 mph before you graduate to jogging. If you're walking at a slower rate, stay with walking. Here are some pointers:

- When you start jogging, do so at a speed no faster than that at which you currently walk.
- As always, warm up and cool down for 5 minutes each. For the warm-up phase, walk briskly and try to gradually raise your heart rate to within at least 20 beats per minute of your target heart rate. On completing your jog, gradually reduce your speed over a 5-minute period to a slow walk.

The box on pages 57-58 shows duration and frequency recommendations for our walk-jog program.

Beginning Stationary Cycling Program

If indoor cycling is more to your liking than walking, that's fine. It's an excellent form of exercise.

Before you begin, you should know your maximal MET value and your weight in either pounds or kilograms. If you haven't had an exercise test to determine your maximal MET value, start out at a comfortable work rate that does not exceed what is recommended for a person with a maximal MET value of 5. Whether you know your maximal MET value or not, I strongly advise against exceeding 75% of your maximal heart rate and an RPE of 13 during these initial weeks. Table 3.3 on page 59 shows your estimated beginning work rate for a stationary cycling program. Choose the body weight closest to yours. Lynne, who weighed 132 lb (60 kg) and had a maximal MET value of 5, began her cycling program at 35 watts. The duration and frequency recommendations for the first 10 weeks of your cycling program are also shown on page 59.

Beginning Schwinn Air-Dyne Cycling Program

A second form of indoor cycling, which works both your arms and legs, is the Schwinn Air-Dyne. The chart for estimating your work load for the first 10 weeks is shown in Table 3.4 on page 60. If you don't know your maximal MET value, start out at a comfortable work load that corresponds to a maximal MET value no higher than 5. Whether you know your maximal MET value or not, I strongly advise against exceeding 75% of your maximal heart rate and an RPE of 13 during these initial weeks. If you weigh 154 pounds (70 kg) and have a maximal MET value of 4, you would see by looking at Table 3.4 that you should begin your Schwinn Air-Dyne cycling program at a work load of 0.6.

The box on page 60 shows the duration and frequency recommendations for your Schwinn Air-Dyne routine. Several other superb cycle ergometers are available that enable you to work your arms and legs simultaneously. Should you prefer to use a different brand, these recommendations are equally applicable.

Beginning Program of Combined Walking and Stationary Cycling Using the Schwinn Air-Dyne

Some people get bored doing the same exercise day after day. For such people, I've devised a 9-week regimen that combines walking with cycling on the Schwinn Air-Dyne. This combination will also help reduce your risk of injury.

The guidelines I've outlined previously for walking and Schwinn Air-Dyne workouts apply. Estimate your starting walking speed and Schwinn Air-Dyne work load for the first 9 weeks of this program using Tables 3.2 and 3.4.

You may start with either activity. As always, warm up for 5 minutes. After completing the first activity, proceed immediately to the other; another warm-up is not needed. Upon completing the second activity, cool down for 5 minutes.

The duration and frequency recommendations for your combined walking and Schwinn Air-Dyne program appear in the box on page 61.

THAT ALL-IMPORTANT TRAINING LOG

I encourage all our stroke patients to keep track of their exercise efforts, at least in the beginning, via a training log. A diary is a good idea because it provides you and your doctor with helpful data. It also will help you be consistent and stay on track with your exercise program. I suggest that you make a number of photocopies of the log on page 55 and put them in a loose-leaf notebook. Fill in a page after each day's exercise:

DAILY EXERCISE TRAINING LOG

Date _____ Time of day _____ Body weight _____

Where I worked out _____

Resting pulse _____

Resting blood pressure (if measured) _____

Post-exercise blood pressure (if measured) _____

Duration of range-of-motion, stretching, & muscle-
   strengthening portion of my workout _____

Pulse rate after range-of-motion, stretching, & muscle-
   strengthening portion of my workout
   (in beats per minute) _____

Aerobic workout

   Type of exercise _____

   Duration (in minutes) _____

   Distance covered or work rate/load _____

   Highest heart rate during workout: _____

   Borg RPE (at most intense part of workout) _____

   Any symptoms experienced _____

Enjoyment rating _____ 1 Very unenjoyable

   _____ 2 Unenjoyable

   _____ 3 Somewhat unenjoyable

   _____ 4 Enjoyable

   _____ 5 Very enjoyable

Health points earned (see chapter 4) _____

Table 3.2
Estimated Speed at Which to Begin a Walking Program

Maximal MET value	Estimated walking speed (miles per hour)	Estimated walking speed (kilometers per hour)
3	1.0 mph	1.6 kph
4	1.8 mph	2.9 kph
5	2.6 mph	4.2 kph
6	3.4 mph	5.4 kph
7 and above	4 mph	6.4 kph

Walking Program		
Week	**Duration per session**	**Frequency per week**
1	2.5 minutes	3-5 times
2	5 minutes	3-5 times
3	7.5 minutes	3-5 times
4	10 minutes	3-5 times
5	12.5 minutes	3-5 times
6	15 minutes	3-5 times
7	20 minutes	3-5 times
8	25 minutes	3-5 times
9	30 minutes	3-5 times
10	35 minutes	3-5 times
11	40 minutes	3-5 times
12	45 minutes	3-5 times
13 and onward	It's time to start earning those 50 to 100 health points a week. Keep your exercise time at 45 minutes per session and gradually increase your speed until you exceed 60% of your maximal heart rate (if you are not doing so yet). If this does not result in the desired weekly energy expenditure using the health points charts in chapter 4,* do one or more of the following: Try exercising within the upper range of your target heart rate zone, exercise more frequently, or increase the duration of each exercise session.	

*At fast speeds, the energy you expend for walking approaches that for jogging. Therefore, for speeds of 4 mph (or 6.4 kph) or faster, I recommend that you use our jogging chart in chapter 4 to calculate your health points.

Walk-Jog Program		
Week	**Duration per session**	**Frequency per week**
1	*20 minutes total—* Walk 4.5 min, jog 0.5 min, walk 4.5 min, jog 0.5 min, walk 4.5 min, jog 0.5 min, walk 4.5 min, jog 0.5 min*	3-5 times
2	*20 minutes total—* Walk 4 min, jog 1 min, walk 4 min, jog 1 min, walk 4 min, jog 1 min, walk 4 min, jog 1 min*	3-5 times
3	*20 minutes total—* Walk 3 min, jog 2 min, walk 3 min, jog 2 min, walk 3 min, jog 2 min, walk 3 min, jog 2 min*	3-5 times
4	*20 minutes total—* Walk 2 min, jog 3 min, walk 2 min, jog 3 min, walk 2 min, jog 3 min, walk 2 min, jog 3 min*	3-5 times
5	*20 minutes total—* Walk 5 min, jog 5 min, walk 5 min, jog 5 min*	3-5 times
6	*20 minutes total—* Walk 4 min, jog 6 min, walk 4 min, jog 6 min*	3-5 times
7	*20 minutes total—* Walk 3 min, jog 7 min, walk 3 min, jog 7 min*	3-5 times

(Cont.)

Walk-Jog Program (Continued)		
Week	**Duration per session**	**Frequency per week**
8	*20 minutes total*—Jog 10 min, walk 10 min*	3-5 times
9	*20 minutes total*—Jog 12 min, walk 8 min*	3-5 times
10	*20 minutes total*—Jog 15 min, walk 5 min*	3-5 times
11	*20 minutes total*—Jog 17 min, walk 3 min*	3-5 times
12	*20 minutes total*—Jog 20 min*	3-5 times
13 and onward	By the time you reach this point, you are likely to have exceeded 60% of your maximal heart rate, and you've possibly attained your desired weekly energy expenditure—100 health points per week —using the health points charts in chapter 4. If so, just keep following week 12's regimen. If, on the other hand, you haven't been able to exceed 60% of your maximal heart rate, increase your speed. If that does not result in 100 weekly health points, do one or more of the following: Try exercising within the upper range of your target heart rate zone, exercise more frequently, or increase the duration of each exercise session.	

*You may find that you are below your desired weekly energy expenditure during the early weeks of this walk-jog effort. You can compensate by walking longer at the end of the jogging phase, before starting your cool-down. Use the jogging chart in chapter 4 when calculating your health points for your walk-jog program.

Table 3.3
**Estimated Work Rate at Which to Begin
a Stationary Cycling (Legs Only) Program**

Maximal MET value	Work rate (watts)					
	Body weight = 110 lb (50 kg)	Body weight = 132 lb (60 kg)	Body weight = 154 lb (70 kg)	Body weight = 176 lb (80 kg)	Body weight = 198 lb (90 kg)	Body weight = 220 lb (100 kg)
3	12	14	16	19	21	23
4	20	25	29	33	37	41
5	29	35	41	47	53	58
6	38	46	53	61	68	76
7	47	56	65	75	84	93
8 and above	55	67	78	89	100	111

Stationary Cycling Program		
Week	**Duration per session**	**Frequency per week**
1	2.5 minutes	3-5 times
2	5 minutes	3-5 times
3	7.5 minutes	3-5 times
4	10 minutes	3-5 times
5	12.5 minutes	3-5 times
6	15 minutes	3-5 times
7	17.5 minutes	3-5 times
8	20 minutes	3-5 times
9	25 minutes	3-5 times
10	30 minutes	3-5 times
11 and onward	It's time to start earning those 50 to 100 health points a week. Keep your exercise time at 30 minutes per session and gradually increase your work rate until you exceed 60% of your maximal heart rate (if you are not doing so yet). If this does not result in the desired weekly energy expenditure using the health points charts in chapter 4, do one or more of the following: Try exercising within the upper range of your target heart rate zone, exercise more frequently, or increase the duration of each exercise session.	

Table 3.4

**Estimated Work Load at Which to Begin
a Schwinn Air-Dyne Cycling Program**

	Work load					
Maximal MET value	Body weight = 110 lb (50 kg)	Body weight = 132 lb (60 kg)	Body weight = 154 lb (70 kg)	Body weight = 176 lb (80 kg)	Body weight = 198 lb (90 kg)	Body weight = 220 lb (100 kg)
3	.2	.3	.4	.4	.4	.5
4	.4	.5	.6	.7	.7	.8
5	.6	.7	.8	.9	1.1	1.2
6	.8	.9	1.1	1.2	1.4	1.5
7	.9	1.1	1.3	1.5	1.7	1.9
8 and above	1.1	1.3	1.6	1.8	2.0	2.2

Schwinn Air-Dyne Program		
Week	**Duration per session**	**Frequency per week**
1	2.5 minutes	3-5 times
2	5 minutes	3-5 times
3	7.5 minutes	3-5 times
4	10 minutes	3-5 times
5	12.5 minutes	3-5 times
6	15 minutes	3-5 times
7	17.5 minutes	3-5 times
8	20 minutes	3-5 times
9	25 minutes	3-5 times
10	30 minutes	3-5 times
11 and onward	It's time to start earning those 50 to 100 health points a week. Keep your exercise time at 30 minutes per session and gradually increase your work load until you exceed 60% of your maximal heart rate (if you are not doing so yet). If this does not result in the desired weekly energy expenditure using the health points charts in chapter 4, do one or more of the following: Try exercising within the upper range of your target heart rate zone, exercise more frequently, or increase the duration of each exercise session.	

Combined Walking and Schwinn Air-Dyne Program

| Week | Duration per session | | Frequency per week |
	Walking	Schwinn Air-Dyne	
1	2.5 minutes	2.5 minutes	3-5 times
2	5 minutes	5 minutes	3-5 times
3	7.5 minutes	7.5 minutes	3-5 times
4	10 minutes	10 minutes	3-5 times
5	12.5 minutes	12.5 minutes	3-5 times
6	15 minutes	15 minutes	3-5 times
7	17.5 minutes	17.5 minutes	3-5 times
8	20 minutes	20 minutes	3-5 times
9	22.5 minutes	22.5 minutes	3-5 times
10 and onward	It's time to start earning those 50 to 100 health points a week. Keep the combined exercise time at 45 minutes per session and gradually increase the intensity until you exceed 60% of your maximal heart rate (if you're not doing so yet). If this does not result in the desired weekly energy expenditure using the health points charts in chapter 4, do one or more of the following: Try exercising within the upper range of your target heart rate zone, exercise more frequently, or increase the duration of each exercise session.		

Chapter 3
Prescription

☐ Start your exercise program slowly and progress gradually, as your condition permits.

☐ Always include both a warm-up and a cool-down of at least 5 minutes in each exercise session.

☐ Do stretching and, unless contraindicated, aerobic exercises three to five times a week.

☐ Include muscle-strengthening exercises in your exercise routines two to three times a week.

☐ Structure the aerobic portion of your workout so that it is eventually 15 to 60 minutes long.

☐ Aim for an exercise intensity that raises your heart rate to between 60% and 75% of your maximal value and elicits an RPE of 12 to 13 during the aerobic portion of your workout.

☐ Don't exceed 85% of your maximal heart rate or an RPE of 15 at any point in your workout.

☐ Make use of interval training to lessen fatigue during exercise if necessary.

☐ Exercise your options: Choose aerobic activities that are convenient to perform.

☐ Keep track of your exercise efforts in a training diary.

Chapter 4

The Health Points System: Insuring Maximum Health Benefits With Minimum Risk

In trying to motivate our stroke patients to follow my exercise prescription, I always feel I'm walking several fine lines. First, as a physician, I have to educate patients adequately so their excuse can never be "I didn't understand." Then I have to alert them to the seriousness of their condition and the risks involved in exercise without leaving them with the feeling it's hopeless. And, most importantly, I have to make them understand that drugs and medical care can only go so far in making them well. They must do the rest by making positive lifestyle changes, including following a regular exercise program.

The impetus for our Health Points System grew out of these needs, especially the need to make you, the patient, responsible for your own health. With our Health Points System, you can chart how effective your exercise program is likely to be in promoting your health.

Our Health Points System was designed so that patients will do just enough exercise to gain optimal health benefits without exerting themselves to the point where exercise increases health risks. Our system gives you, the stroke patient, a way to strike a balance between the twin goals of effectiveness and safety.

HOW THE HEALTH POINTS SYSTEM WORKS

Our system is based on the number of calories people should expend during exercise, which varies according to weight. In chapter 3, I discussed what doctors and exercise physiologists have learned about aerobic exercise and its effect on health. Let's review this key finding:

Aerobic exercise performed for 15 to 60 minutes per workout 3 to 5 days each week at an intensity that raises the heart rate to between 60% and 85% of the maximal value will result in an energy expenditure that brings about the desired health benefits.

Here's how our Health Points System works. If you're a novice exerciser, consider following one of the beginning exercise programs outlined in chapter 3, and gradually work your body up to an appropriate level of exertion over 10 to 12 weeks or so. Although you can start using the Weekly Health Points Exercise Tally Sheet (see page 65) during this time, you should not specifically try to earn 50 to 100 health points weekly until you reach Weeks 10 to 12. Depending on the extent of your disability, it may take you longer than this—even months—to earn the desired number of points. That's fine. Be patient.

In all aspects of life, we humans like to know where we stand in our endeavors. We like to get report cards. Our Health Points System is like a report card on your exercise program. Only you fill it out, not a doctor or a teacher. Our Health Points System enables you to quantify one constructive lifestyle change (namely, regular aerobic exercise) you can easily make to improve your health (and reduce your risk for a repeat stroke and other serious chronic diseases). It gives you a way to chart your progress so you can see, in black and white, what you have accomplished.

I must remind you that our Health Points System is primarily intended for those of you with no disability or only a slight one. While many with a moderate disability will also be able to use it, it's definitely not intended for anyone with a more severe disability.

WEEKLY HEALTH POINTS EXERCISE TALLY SHEET

Your Weekly Goal: To earn between 50 and 100 health points each week, which corresponds to an expenditure of 10 to 20 calories per kilogram (2.2 pounds) of body weight per week. Exceeding this upper limit does not provide substantially more health benefit; thus you should keep your weekly health points total at, or very near, 100. To gain optimal benefit, you should earn your weekly quota of points across at least 3 workouts.

To find out how many health points you earned during an exercise session, simply use the chart (see Tables 4.1-4.5, pages 77-84) that corresponds to the form of aerobic exercise you're doing and fill in the results below:

Monday	Tuesday	Wednesday	Thursday	Friday	Saturday	Sunday		Total weekly health points
___ pt. +	___ pt. +	___ pt. +	___ pt. +	___ pt. +	___ pt. +	___ pt.	=	___ pt. (100 pt. maximum)

INTERPRETING THE EFFECTIVENESS OF YOUR WEEKLY EXERCISE EFFORT*

100 health points from exercise	Ideal. *You couldn't do better!*
70-99 health points from exercise	Very good. *Be proud of yourself.*
50-69 health points from exercise	Good. *But you could do better.*
20-49 health points from exercise	Fair. *Try a bit harder.*
10-19 health points from exercise	Poor. *But it's better than nothing.*
Less than 10 health points from exercise	Very poor. *Come on, now.*

*If your medical condition is such that you cannot attain the desired weekly number of health points, ignore this interpretation. Be proud of whatever progress you are able to make.

If you have no disability or only a slight one (see chapter 2), your goal should be to earn as close to 100 health points a week as possible. Those of you with anything more than a slight disability, though, should be satisfied with 50 health points per week.

If your physical condition prevents you from attaining the desired weekly number of health points, don't worry or become discouraged. If you perform some aerobic exercise—even an exercise for which I don't provide health points charts—for a minimum of 15 minutes at least 3 days a week, your health will benefit. Rather than trying to meet goals that may be unrealistic at present, be proud of what progress you do make. Also, keep in mind that the effectiveness categories on the weekly tally sheet are not applicable to persons whose disability (as opposed to factors such as a lack of interest or desire) prevents them from attaining the recommended number of weekly health points.

HOW TO USE
THE HEALTH POINTS CHARTS

The only way to get an accurate reading of energy expenditure during exercise is through laboratory testing. There, technicians use sophisticated equipment to measure the exact amount of oxygen the body uses during a workout. The charts that follow are derived from numerous exercise research studies performed in such laboratories.

The health points charts found at the end of this chapter (Tables 4.1-4.4) cover walking, jogging, stationary cycling (legs only), and the Schwinn Air-Dyne—all of which were described in chapter 3. It was possible to formulate charts for these forms of exercise because (a) none require much skill and (b) outstanding research data are available for them.

The charts are designed for stroke patients with no more than a slight to moderate impairment in ability to use the affected leg.[1,2] If you walk with a limp or use a cane or other assistance aid, including special orthotics, add 15% to your health points score for any weight-bearing activities that you do. (To add 15%, simply multiply your health points score by 1.15.)

If you're exercising on equipment that I have not provided charts for but that gives you a readout of the number of calories you've expended, you can easily convert such a number to health points. First, divide your body weight in pounds by 11 (or if your body weight is in kilograms, divide it by 5) to obtain your conversion factor. Then divide the readout number by that factor to obtain your health points.

For example, if the readout number is 120 calories and you weigh 165 pounds (75 kilograms), you've earned 8 health points (165/11 = 75/5 = 15 and 120 calories/15 = 8 health points).

To determine the health points you earn for walking and jogging, you need to know the distance you covered during your workout (to convert kilometers to miles, divide by 1.6) and the time it took you. If you're lucky enough to have access to a measured running track, figuring the distance will pose no problem. Otherwise you might want to invest in a pedometer or use your car's odometer to stake out a stretch of road to use as a track. You'll need a watch with a second hand or a stopwatch to accurately measure the duration of your session.

To find your health points on the charts for stationary cycling and the Schwinn Air-Dyne, you'll need to know the duration of your workout, your work rate (wattage) or work load (for the Schwinn Air-Dyne), and your weight (to convert kilograms to pounds, multiply by 2.2).

I have not provided charts for wheelchair locomotion because special ones aren't necessary. Wheelchair locomotion expends about the same energy as normal walking, so use that chart to figure your health points score.[2] If your speed is 4 mph (6.4 kph) or faster, use our jogging chart instead.

To show you how easy the Health Points System is to use, on pages 68 and 69 are some examples from Roger's training diary. At the time of Week A, which was 10 weeks into his training program, Roger weighed 198 pounds (about 90 kilograms). During Week B, some 6 months later, his weight was down to 176 pounds (80 kilograms) due to his improved eating and exercising habits.

These workouts during Week A enabled Roger to earn 34 health points, somewhat below our recommended goal of at least 50 health points per week.

This schedule for Week B enabled Roger to earn 80 health points, close to our optimal weekly recommended goal of 100 health points.

OTHER AEROBIC CHOICES: THE PROS AND CONS

To vary your routine, you may want to try some other forms of exercise. When doing so, keep in mind that these other forms of aerobic exercise require considerable skill, are influenced by external factors such as the weather or terrain, or have not been adequately researched. Table 4.5 shows you how to figure your health points

Week A

Date	Activity	Time	Distance/ work load	Health points	Notes
S					
M	Walk	22-1/2 min	.9 miles	6	*Walking felt good.*
	Schwinn Air-Dyne	22 min	.6 WL	5.7	
T					
W	Walk	15 min	.6 miles	4.1	*Planned to walk 22 min, but*
	Cycle (legs)	25 min	40 watts	7	*had to stop after 15.*
T					
F	Walk	20 min	.8 miles	5.7	*Good workout.*
	Schwinn Air-Dyne	20 min	.7 WL	5.2	
S					
				34	**Total: Week** *10*

for other aerobic activities. This table is very useful, but it isn't as precise as the charts for walking, jogging, and stationary cycling. To use this table, you need to know how long you exercised and whether you exercised at a light (RPE < 12), moderate (RPE = 12-13), or heavy (RPE > 13) intensity.

Week B

Date	Activity	Time	Distance/ work load	Health points	Notes
S					
M	Walk	20 min	1.1 miles	6.5	Good walk.
	Schwinn Air-Dyne	20 min	1.5 WL	9.2	
T	Walk	40 min	2 miles	12.5	Nice day for a walk.
W	Walk	25 min	1.4 miles	8.2	Legs felt weak today.
	Cycle (legs)	20 min	60 watts	7.6	
T					
F	Exercise class	30 min	12 RPE	15.9	I like exercising with others.
	Schwinn Air-Dyne	15 min	1.5 WL	6.9	
S	Swim	30 min	13.2 RPE	13.2	Tough to get in 30 minutes.
				80	**Total: Week** 36

The ideal aerobic exercise for you has three basic characteristics:

- It's pleasant. An exercise you enjoy is one you're more likely to stick with.
- It's practical and it fits into your lifestyle. In short, it's something you can do conveniently year-round.

- It uses large muscle groups. The larger the muscle groups you exercise, the greater your body's oxygen uptake (and hence energy expenditure) will be.

Here are the pros and cons of some other aerobic exercise choices:

Swimming

This is an excellent aerobic activity because it uses both upper and lower body muscles. And, because it's a non-weight-bearing activity, the chances of a musculoskeletal injury are extremely low. Moreover, the warmth of the water may help relax you and relieve any stiffness in your body. Swimming is especially valuable for people with lower back problems, arthritis, heat-regulation disorders, or balance problems.

Swimming—and other forms of water exercise—are among the best aerobic choices for people who have had strokes. But for many people, swimming is not an option. It requires a pool and the means to get there at the right hours. This is the only reason I didn't include it in my beginning aerobic exercise choices in chapter 3.

The normal recommended pool temperature is 86 °F (30 °C). Temperatures should not exceed 100 °F (about 38 °C) because this reduces your capacity to perform aerobic exercise and may trigger cardiovascular problems.[3]

Aqua-Aerobics

This is just what the name implies—aerobic exercises (including walking) done in water. The pros and cons of this increasingly popular low-impact activity are similar to those for swimming. Those of you who find the prospect of exercising in a swimming pool appealing might want to consult Ken Cooper's book *Overcoming Hypertension* for detailed guidelines.[4]

Cross-Country Skiing

Ken Cooper rates this as the top aerobics activity because "you have more muscles involved than just the legs; and any time you get more muscles involved, you get more aerobic benefit."[5] In addition, the added weight of clothing and equipment further enhances the aerobic effect (that is, your energy expenditure) over that of walking or jogging at similar speeds.

There are drawbacks, though. The total exertion is greatly affected by variations in skill, snow surface, terrain, temperature and weather conditions, and altitude. Also, it's difficult to take your pulse in the middle of this activity. One way around these barriers is to use cross-country skiing machines. For stroke patients who have the functional ability to use them, I am enthusiastic about this equipment. Exercising on such equipment enables you to burn calories in a highly efficient manner, and it's also unlikely to cause musculoskeletal problems.

Stair Climbing

A testament to the current popularity of stair-climbing machines is that they always seem to be in use at health clubs. These machines simulate the act of climbing flights of stairs, thus enabling you to work the large muscles in your back, buttocks, and legs and to expend lots of energy quickly. But stair climbing is strenuous and may cause a rapid rise in heart rate and blood pressure, so it's generally not appropriate for beginners. If the idea of stair climbing appeals to you, wait until you've been working out for at least 12 weeks before adding it to your exercise regimen.[6]

People with knee problems should probably avoid stair climbing, for the stress it places on the knee joint is thought to be equivalent to lifting four to six times your body weight.[6] It's likely to aggravate existing problems in that area.

Rope Skipping

This is a practical, enjoyable, and easily accessible aerobic activity. But it's not a popular choice because it involves a lot of skill, is relatively strenuous, and may result in excessively high heart rates. Even at that, for a given heart rate, the energy expenditure is not as high as that for some other strenuous aerobic exercises, such as jogging. Rope skipping does, however, expose you to the risk of musculoskeletal disorders; this is a significant drawback.

Aerobic Dance

Aerobic dancing involves steady, rhythmic movements done to the beat of relatively fast music, usually rock. Recently, benches that range in height from 6 to 12 inches (15 to 30 cm) have been introduced into aerobic dance workouts to increase the exercise intensity while reducing the impact and risk of injury. But I do not recommend aerobic dance for most stroke patients, especially those with heart disease, unless the class is specifically designed for them (and, frankly, I don't know of many). Aerobic dancing is strenuous and will probably cause you to exceed your training heart rate limit.

Circuit Resistance Training

This is a combination of aerobics and muscle strengthening. Typically an exerciser would use a series of resistance-training machines and move from one to the next with very short rest periods (15 to 30 seconds) in between. Performed correctly, circuit training improves the cardiovascular system, builds and tones muscles, and burns calories during one carefully constructed workout.

Sounds great, doesn't it?

I didn't want to dismiss this exercise option out of hand, so I reviewed the medical literature and did my own study of its possible rehabilitation benefits.[7] Here's the catch: The primary benefit is enhancement of muscular strength, not energy expenditure. Also, it may cause an excessive rise in blood pressure.

So it's best for stroke patients to avoid circuit resistance training unless they've got appropriate medical supervision and guidance. Even then, it should still be performed in combination with other more traditional forms of aerobic exercise. And remember to adhere to the muscle-strengthening guidelines in chapter 3.

Recreational Sports

If you have only a slight disability, you can participate in many recreational sports. But you should be aware that once activities turn competitive, the risk of cardiovascular complications goes up. If you engage in recreational sports, you may have to modify the rules to minimize the competitive aspects so you can keep your heart rate within the designated limits. When performed in such a way, recreational sports can be, and often are, a valuable part of a stroke rehabilitation exercise program.

Although I have not included sample introductory programs for each of these alternative exercise choices, you can use the walking and stationary cycling programs at the end of chapter 3 as prototypes for your own programs. For example, an introductory swimming program might be as follows:

Week	Duration per session	Frequency per week
1	2.5 minutes	3-5 times
2	5 minutes	3-5 times
3	7.5 minutes	3-5 times
4	10 minutes	3-5 times
5	12.5 minutes	3-5 times
6	15 minutes	3-5 times
7	17.5 minutes	3-5 times
8	20 minutes	3-5 times
9	25 minutes	3-5 times
10	30 minutes	3-5 times
11 and onward	It's time to start earning those 50 to 100 health points a week. Keep your exercise time at 30 minutes per session and gradually increase your swimming speed until you exceed 60% of your maximal heart rate (if you are not doing so yet). If this does not result in the desired weekly energy expenditure using the Other Aerobic Activities chart (Table 4.5, pp. 82-84), do one or more of the following: Try exercising within the upper range of your target heart rate zone, exercise more frequently, or increase the duration of each exercise session.	

In using this swimming program, as with any aerobic exercise, begin at a comfortable intensity. During the initial weeks you would not exceed 75% of your maximal heart rate and an RPE of 13. Be sure to warm up and cool down for at least 5 minutes each. You can do this by swimming at a slower pace or doing other activities in the water.

THE FOUR-LETTER WORD
YOU MUST NOT UTTER

That word is *quit*.

You've probably noticed I keep pushing the notion of *regular* exercise—not sporadic exercise, not fair-weather exercise, but the kind

Other aerobic choices

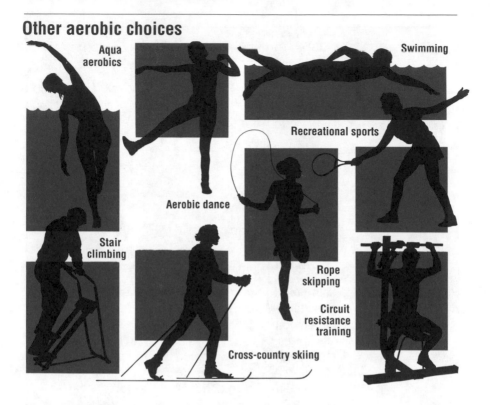

Aqua aerobics

Swimming

Recreational sports

Aerobic dance

Stair climbing

Rope skipping

Circuit resistance training

Cross-country skiing

of persistent exercise you engage in almost daily because it's a habit, like brushing your teeth. There's a reason. When you exercise, your body and its organ systems are exposed to potent physiological stimuli. If you exercise regularly at an appropriate intensity and duration, these stimuli cause specific adaptations that both enhance your ability to exercise and improve your health. In other words, you'll receive all the benefits of a physically active lifestyle (benefits I outlined in chapter 2).

But you can't store these benefits for a rainy day. They're reversible. All it takes to set this backtracking in motion is abstinence. If you stop training or reduce your physical activity below your required level, your body's systems soon readjust themselves to this diminished amount of physiological stimuli. And those hard-won, exercise-related gains, which you worked so long and hard to achieve, are lost.

This *reversibility concept* is best summed up by a landmark study of 16,936 Harvard University alumni by Ralph S. Paffenbarger, Jr., and his colleagues.[8] In this study, many former college athletes became inactive adults. Consequently, they were in worse shape—and at greater risk for cardiovascular disease—than their contemporaries who had not participated in college sports but who had started exercising later in life. Researchers do not know how long it takes after you stop training before all the health benefits of exercise are lost. We do know that even after many years of training, a rapid decline in fitness occurs during the first 12 to 21 days of inactivity—and the fitness benefits of regular exercise are almost totally lost after about 2 or 3 months.[9]

So it's vital that you stick with your exercise program once you get started. But this is easier said than done. Several studies on exercise compliance found that half or more of all patients drop out of their exercise programs within 6 months; the critical dropout period is the first 3 months or so. To get through this critical time, you need motivators. The following suggestions will keep you huffing and puffing even when you'd rather be home in bed or watching television.

• *Make sure you fully understand the costs of not exercising versus the benefits of exercising.*

• *Start exercising slowly and progress gradually.* If you follow the beginning programs outlined in this book, you'll be doing just that.

Exercise dropout rate

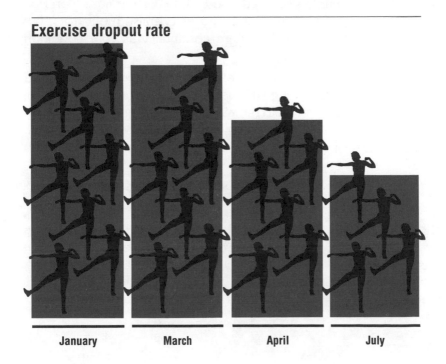

| January | March | April | July |

• *Choose a form of exercise that's convenient as well as enjoyable.* If you constantly score below a "4" on the enjoyment rating checklist in the exercise log (at the end of chapter 3), your exercise program needs to be modified.

• *Find a role model*—a friend, relative, or acquaintance who leads a physically active life. Find out why he or she loves exercise.

• *Learn from your past exercise experiences.* Try to figure out where you went wrong previously.

• *Obtain as much support for your exercise program as possible.* Enlist the company—or, at the very least, the moral support—of those closest to you. Health promotion should be a family affair. After all, your relatives are also at risk for having a stroke or developing such conditions as heart disease. Explain this to your family, and use it as the rationale to get as many of them as possible involved in your exercise program. In more ways than one, you're all in this together.

Seek the support of others, but never let peer pressure force you to exercise more strenuously than you should. Although exercising with others has many advantages, always work at your own pace. You've got a special condition—you've had a stroke—and even if your exercise companion has had one too, his or her case won't be the same as yours. Goals are important as exercise motivators, but keep yours realistic and modify them continually as your condition changes.

• *Bring your body to your place of exercise, even if your mind is temporarily on strike.* Often it's just a matter of overcoming mental inertia. A body at rest prefers to remain at rest, no doubt. But once you start exercising, you may find you enjoy it more than you anticipated. Remember, special occasions, such as holidays or vacations, are no excuse.

• *Finally, remember that exercise is forever.* Make physical activity a lifelong pursuit.

Don't be an exercise dropout. I urge you to do everything in your power to stick with your exercise program, especially during the crucial initial months. Once you've passed the 6-month mark and tasted the tantalizing benefits of an active lifestyle, I think there's less and less chance you'll ever revert back to your old unhealthy inactivity.

Table 4.1
Walking Health Points Chart

Time (min:sec)	Distance (miles)	Health points	Time (min:sec)	Distance (miles)	Health points
5:00	Under 0.10	0.8	7:30	Under 0.15	1.3
	0.10-0.14	1.0		0.15-0.19	1.5
	0.15-0.19	1.2		0.20-0.24	1.7
	0.20-0.24	1.4		0.25-0.29	1.9
	0.25-0.29	1.6		0.30-0.34	2.1
	0.30-0.33	1.8		0.35-0.39	2.3
	Over 0.33	*		0.40-0.44	2.5
				0.45-0.49	2.7
				Over 0.49	*
10:00	Under 0.20	1.7	12:30	Under 0.20	1.9
	0.20-0.24	1.8		0.20-0.29	2.3
	0.25-0.29	2.0		0.30-0.39	2.7
	0.30-0.34	2.2		0.40-0.49	3.1
	0.35-0.39	2.4		0.50-0.59	3.5
	0.40-0.44	2.6		0.60-0.69	3.9
	0.45-0.49	2.8		0.70-0.79	4.3
	0.50-0.54	3.0		0.80-0.83	4.7
	0.55-0.59	3.2		Over 0.83	*
	0.60-0.66	3.6			
	Over 0.66	*			
15:00	Under 0.30	2.5	17:30	Under 0.30	2.8
	0.30-0.39	2.9		0.30-0.49	3.5
	0.40-0.49	3.3		0.50-0.69	4.3
	0.50-0.59	3.7		0.70-0.89	5.1
	0.60-0.69	4.1		0.90-1.09	5.9
	0.70-0.79	4.5		1.10-1.16	6.7
	0.80-0.89	4.9		Over 1.16	*
	0.90-0.99	5.3			
	Over 0.99	*			
20:00	Under 0.40	3.4	22:30	Under 0.40	3.6
	0.40-0.59	4.1		0.40-0.59	4.4
	0.60-0.79	4.9		0.60-0.79	5.2
	0.80-0.99	5.7		0.80-0.99	6.0
	1.00-1.19	6.5		1.00-1.19	6.8
	1.20-1.33	7.3		1.20-1.39	7.6
	Over 1.33	*		1.40-1.49	8.4
				Over 1.49	*
25:00	Under 0.50	4.2	27:30	Under 0.50	4.5
	0.50-0.69	5.0		0.50-0.69	5.2
	0.70-0.89	5.8		0.70-0.89	6.0

(Cont.)

Table 4.1
Continued

Time (min:sec)	Distance (miles)	Health points	Time (min:sec)	Distance (miles)	Health points
25:00 (Cont.)			27:30 (Cont.)		
	0.90-1.09	6.6		0.90-1.09	6.8
	1.10-1.29	7.4		1.10-1.29	7.6
	1.30-1.49	8.2		1.30-1.49	8.4
	1.50-1.66	9.0		1.50-1.69	9.2
	Over 1.66	*		1.70-1.83	10.0
				Over 1.83	*
30:00	Under 0.50	4.6	35:00	Under 0.75	6.1
	0.50-0.74	5.6		0.75-0.99	7.0
	0.75-0.99	6.6		1.00-1.24	8.0
	1.00-1.24	7.6		1.25-1.49	9.0
	1.25-1.49	8.6		1.50-1.74	10.0
	1.50-1.74	9.6		1.75-1.99	11.0
	1.75-1.99	10.6		2.00-2.24	12.0
	Over 1.99	*		2.25-2.33	13.0
				Over 2.33	*
40:00	Under 1.00	7.5	45:00	Under 1.00	7.9
	1.00-1.24	8.5		1.00-1.49	9.9
	1.25-1.49	9.5		1.50-1.99	11.9
	1.50-1.74	10.5		2.00-2.49	13.9
	1.75-1.99	11.5		2.50-2.99	15.9
	2.00-2.24	12.5		Over 2.99	*
	2.25-2.49	13.5			
	2.50-2.66	14.5			
	Over 2.66	*			
50:00	Under 1.00	8.4	55:00	Under 1.00	8.8
	1.00-1.49	10.3		1.00-1.49	10.8
	1.50-1.99	12.4		1.50-1.99	12.8
	2.00-2.49	14.4		2.00-2.49	14.8
	2.50-2.99	16.4		2.50-2.99	16.8
	3.00-3.33	18.4		3.00-3.49	18.8
	Over 3.33	*		3.50-3.66	20.8
				Over 3.66	*
60:00	Under 1.00	9.3			
	1.00-1.49	11.2			
	1.50-1.99	13.2			
	2.00-2.49	15.2			
	2.50-2.99	17.2			
	3.00-3.49	19.2			
	3.50-3.99	21.2			
	Over 3.99	*			

*Use the Jogging Health Points Chart (Table 4.2).

Table 4.2
Jogging Health Points Chart

Time (min:sec)	Distance (miles)	Health points	Time (min:sec)	Distance (miles)	Health points
5:00	Under 0.40	3.6	7:30	Under 0.50	4.7
	0.40-0.49	4.4		0.50-0.59	5.4
	0.50-0.59	5.2		0.60-0.69	6.2
	0.60-0.69	6.0		0.70-0.79	7.0
	Over 0.69	6.8		0.80-0.89	7.8
				0.90-0.99	8.6
				1.00-1.09	9.4
				Over 1.09	10.2
10:00	Under 0.80	7.3	12:30	Under 1.00	9.2
	0.80-0.89	8.0		1.00-1.19	10.7
	0.90-0.99	8.8		1.20-1.39	12.3
	1.00-1.09	9.6		1.40-1.59	13.9
	1.10-1.19	10.4		1.60-1.79	15.5
	1.20-1.29	11.2		Over 1.79	17.1
	1.30-1.39	12.0			
	1.40-1.49	12.8			
	Over 1.49	13.6			
15:00	Under 1.20	10.9	17:30	Under 1.40	12.8
	1.20-1.39	12.5		1.40-1.59	14.3
	1.40-1.59	14.1		1.60-1.79	15.9
	1.60-1.79	15.7		1.80-1.99	17.5
	1.80-1.99	17.3		2.00-2.19	19.1
	2.00-2.19	18.9		2.20-2.39	20.7
	Over 2.19	20.5		2.40-2.59	22.4
				Over 2.59	24.0
20:00	Under 1.50	13.8	22:30	Under 1.75	16.0
	1.50-1.74	15.7		1.75-1.99	18.0
	1.75-1.99	17.7		2.00-2.24	20.0
	2.00-2.24	19.7		2.25-2.49	22.0
	2.25-2.49	21.7		2.50-2.74	24.0
	2.50-2.74	23.7		2.75-2.99	26.0
	2.75-2.99	25.7		3.00-3.24	28.0
	Over 2.99	27.7		Over 3.24	30.0
25:00	Under 2.00	18.2	27:30	Under 2.00	18.5
	2.00-2.24	20.2		2.00-2.24	20.4
	2.25-2.49	22.2		2.25-2.49	22.4
	2.50-2.74	24.2		2.50-2.74	24.4
	2.75-2.99	26.2		2.75-2.99	26.4
	3.00-3.24	28.2		3.00-3.24	28.4
	3.25-3.49	30.2		3.25-3.49	30.4

(Cont.)

Table 4.2
Continued

Time (min:sec)	Distance (miles)	Health points	Time (min:sec)	Distance (miles)	Health points
25:00 (Cont.)			27:30 (Cont.)		
	3.50-3.74	32.2		3.50-3.74	32.5
	Over 3.74	34.2		3.75-3.99	34.5
				Over 3.99	36.5
30:00	Under 2.50	22.7	35:00	Under 2.75	25.1
	2.50-2.74	24.6		2.75-2.99	27.0
	2.75-2.99	26.6		3.00-3.24	29.1
	3.00-3.24	28.6		3.25-3.49	31.1
	3.25-3.49	30.6		3.50-3.74	33.1
	3.50-3.74	32.6		3.75-3.99	35.1
	3.75-3.99	34.6		4.00-4.24	37.1
	4.00-4.24	36.6		4.25-4.49	39.1
	Over 4.24	38.6		4.50-4.74	41.1
				4.75-4.99	43.1
				Over 4.99	45.1
40:00	Under 3.00	27.6	45:00	Under 3.50	32.0
	3.00-3.49	31.5		3.50-3.99	35.9
	3.50-3.99	35.5		4.00-4.49	40.0
	4.00-4.49	39.5		4.50-4.99	44.0
	4.50-4.99	43.5		5.00-5.49	48.0
	5.00-5.49	47.5		5.50-5.99	52.0
	5.50-5.99	51.6		6.00-6.49	56.0
	Over 5.99	55.6		Over 6.49	60.0
50:00	Under 4.00	36.5	55:00	Under 4.50	40.9
	4.00-4.49	40.4		4.50-4.99	44.8
	4.50-4.99	44.4		5.00-5.49	48.9
	5.00-5.49	48.4		5.50-5.99	52.9
	5.50-5.99	52.4		6.00-6.49	56.9
	6.00-6.49	56.4		6.50-6.99	60.9
	6.50-6.99	60.4		7.00-7.49	64.9
	7.00-7.49	64.5		7.50-7.99	68.9
	Over 7.49	68.5		Over 7.99	72.9
60:00	Under 4.50	41.3			
	4.50-4.99	45.3			
	5.00-5.49	49.3			
	5.50-5.99	53.3			
	6.00-6.49	57.3			
	6.50-6.99	61.3			
	7.00-7.49	65.3			
	7.50-7.99	69.3			
	8.00-8.49	73.4			
	8.50-8.99	77.4			
	Over 8.99	81.4			

Table 4.3
Stationary Cycling (Legs Only) Health Points Chart

Work rate (watts)	Under 100 lb	100 to 124 lb	125 to 149 lb	150 to 174 lb	175 to 199 lb	200 to 224 lb	225 to 249 lb	Over 249 lb
				Health points per minute				
Under 25	0.34	0.28	0.24	0.22	0.20	0.18	0.17	0.16
25-49	0.54	0.44	0.36	0.32	0.28	0.26	0.24	0.22
50-74	0.76	0.60	0.50	0.42	0.38	0.34	0.32	0.30
75-99	0.98	0.76	0.62	0.54	0.48	0.42	0.38	0.36
100-124	1.20	0.92	0.76	0.64	0.56	0.50	0.46	0.42
125-149	1.42	1.10	0.90	0.76	0.66	0.58	0.54	0.48
150-174	1.64	1.26	1.02	0.86	0.76	0.68	0.60	0.56
175-199	1.86	1.42	1.16	0.98	0.84	0.76	0.68	0.62
200-224	2.08	1.58	1.28	1.08	0.94	0.84	0.76	0.68
225-249	2.30	1.76	1.42	1.20	1.04	0.92	0.82	0.76
Over 249	2.52	1.92	1.56	1.30	1.14	1.00	0.90	0.82

Table 4.4
Schwinn Air-Dyne Health Points Chart

Work load	Under 100 lb	100 to 124 lb	125 to 149 lb	150 to 174 lb	175 to 199 lb	200 to 224 lb	225 to 249 lb	Over 249 lb
				Health points per minute				
Under 0.5	0.34	0.28	0.24	0.22	0.20	0.18	0.17	0.16
0.5-0.9	0.52	0.40	0.34	0.30	0.26	0.24	0.22	0.21
1.0-1.4	0.74	0.56	0.48	0.40	0.36	0.32	0.30	0.28
1.5-1.9	0.96	0.74	0.60	0.52	0.46	0.42	0.38	0.34
2.0-2.4	1.18	0.90	0.74	0.62	0.56	0.50	0.44	0.42
2.5-2.9	1.40	1.06	0.86	0.74	0.64	0.58	0.52	0.48
3.0-3.4	1.62	1.22	1.00	0.84	0.74	0.66	0.60	0.54
3.5-3.9	1.84	1.40	1.14	0.96	0.84	0.74	0.66	0.62
4.0-4.4	2.06	1.56	1.26	1.06	0.92	0.82	0.74	0.68
4.5-4.9	2.28	1.72	1.40	1.18	1.02	0.90	0.82	0.74
Over 4.9	2.50	1.88	1.52	1.28	1.12	0.98	0.88	0.80

Table 4.5
Other Aerobic Activities

| Activity | Health points per minute | | |
| | Intensity* | | |
	Light	Moderate	Heavy
Aerobic dancing	0.35	0.53	0.79
Alpine skiing	0.35	0.53	0.70
Aqua-aerobics	0.35	0.53	0.79
Arm-cycle ergometry	0.22	0.35	0.61
Backpacking	0.53	0.70	0.88
(5% slope, 44 lb or 20 kg)			
4.0 mph (6.4 kph)	0.70		
4.5 mph (7.2 kph)	0.84		
5.0 mph (8.0 kph)	1.02		
6.0 mph (9.6 kph)	1.15		
7.0 mph (11.2 kph)	1.36		
Badminton	0.26	0.53	0.79
Ballet	0.44	0.53	0.70
Ballroom dancing	0.26	0.35	0.44
Baseball	0.26	0.35	0.44
Basketball	0.53	0.70	0.96
Bicycling	0.26	0.61	0.88
6.3 mph (10 kph)	0.42		
9.4 mph (15 kph)	0.52		
12.5 mph (20 kph)	0.62		
15.6 mph (25 kph)	0.74		
18.8 mph (30 kph)	0.86		
Canoeing	0.26	0.35	0.53
Catch (ball)	0.26	0.35	0.44
Circuit resistance training	0.26	0.44	0.61
Cricket	0.26	0.35	0.44
Cross-country skiing	0.44	0.79	1.14
2.5 mph (4 kph)	0.48		
3.8 mph (6 kph)	0.67		
5.0 mph (8 kph)	0.87		
6.3 mph (10 kph)	1.07		
7.5 mph (12 kph)	1.25		
8.8 mph (14 kph)	1.44		
Exercise classes	0.35	0.53	0.79
Fencing	0.44	0.61	0.88
Field hockey	0.53	0.70	0.88
Figure skating	0.35	0.53	0.88
Football (American)	0.44	0.53	0.61
Football (touch)	0.44	0.53	0.70

(Cont.)

Table 4.5
(Continued)

| Activity | Health points per minute | | |
| | Intensity* | | |
	Light	Moderate	Heavy
Golf			
Carrying clubs	0.45		
Pulling cart	0.35		
Riding cart	0.22		
Gymnastics	0.44	0.61	0.88
Handball (4-wall)	0.53	0.70	0.96
Hiking	0.26	0.53	0.70
Home calisthenics	0.26	0.44	0.70
Hunting	0.26	0.44	0.61
Ice hockey	0.53	0.70	0.88
Judo	0.53	0.70	1.05
Karate	0.44	0.70	1.05
Kayaking	0.53	0.70	0.96
7.8 mph (12.5 kph)	0.68		
9.4 mph (15.0 kph)	0.96		
Lacrosse	0.53	0.70	0.88
Modern dancing	0.44	0.53	0.70
Mountaineering	0.61	0.70	0.88
Orienteering	0.70	0.88	1.05
Racquetball	0.53	0.79	1.05
Rebounding	0.31	0.44	0.53
Rollerskating	0.44	0.57	0.70
Rope skipping	0.61	0.88	1.05
66 per min	0.86		
84 per min	0.92		
100 per min	0.96		
120 per min	1.00		
125 per min	1.02		
130 per min	1.03		
135 per min	1.05		
145 per min	1.06		
Rowing	0.61	0.88	1.14
2.5 mph (4 kph)	0.48		
5.0 mph (8 kph)	0.90		
7.5 mph (12 kph)	1.18		
10.0 mph (16 kph)	1.44		
12.5 mph (20 kph)	1.67		

(Cont.)

Table 4.5
Continued

| Activity | Health points per minute | | |
| | Intensity* | | |
	Light	Moderate	Heavy
Rugby	0.53	0.70	0.96
Scuba diving	0.35	0.44	0.53
Sculling	0.35	0.53	0.88
Skateboarding	0.44	0.57	0.70
Skating (ice)	0.35	0.61	1.14
11.3 mph (18 kph)	0.35		
15.6 mph (25 kph)	0.42		
17.5 mph (28 kph)	0.81		
20.0 mph (32 kph)	0.95		
22.5 mph (36 kph)	1.33		
Snorkeling	0.35	0.44	0.53
Soccer	0.44	0.61	0.96
Softball	0.26	0.35	0.44
Squash	0.53	0.79	1.05
Stair climbing	0.35	0.61	0.96
Swimming (beach)	0.18	0.26	0.35
Swimming (pool)	0.26	0.44	0.79
1.3 mph (2 kph)	0.38		
1.6 mph (2.5 kph)	0.60		
1.9 mph (3.0 kph)	0.78		
2.2 mph (3.5 kph)	1.01		
2.5 mph (4.0 kph)	1.19		
Synchronized swimming	0.35	0.53	0.70
Table tennis	0.26	0.44	0.70
Tennis	0.35	0.53	0.88
Volleyball	0.44	0.53	0.70
Walking up stairs	0.35	0.53	0.70
Water polo	0.53	0.70	0.96
Wrestling	0.53	0.79	1.05

*Light intensity results in minimal perspiration and only a slight increase in breathing above normal (RPE of less than 12). Moderate intensity results in definite perspiration and above normal breathing (RPE of 12-13). Heavy intensity corresponds to heavy perspiration and breathing (RPE of more than 13). These values are adapted from an expert committee report of the Canada Fitness Survey - source M. Jette et al., Clinical Cardiology, 13 (1990): 555-565.

Chapter 4

Prescription

□ If you're a novice exerciser, consider using one of my beginning exercise programs (see chapter 3). Let your doctor help you adapt it to suit your particular case.

□ Use our Health Points System to gain optimal health benefits with minimal risk.

□ When using our Health Points System, adjust your frequency, intensity, and duration of exercise to earn 50 to 100 points each week.

□ Do not attempt to earn your quota of health points in fewer than three workouts—on at least 3 separate days—each week.

□ Keep your goals realistic and modify them continually.

□ If your physical condition is such that you cannot attain the desired weekly health points, don't become discouraged. If you do some type of aerobic exercise for a minimum of 15 minutes at least 3 days per week, you'll gain important health benefits.

□ Be proud of whatever progress you are able to make.

□ Do everything in your power to keep from becoming an exercise dropout, especially during the crucial initial months.

□ Don't get discouraged! You can do it.

Chapter 5

Staying Within the Safe-Exercise Zone: Essential Exercise Guidelines for Stroke Survivors

Fortunately, prescribing exercise for stroke patients is not the guessing game it was in the past. Today, well-informed physicians can prescribe exercise just as they would medications. However, as with drugs, certain precautions are needed to make sure your exercise plan is both safe and effective.

Even healthy people should follow general safety guidelines when exercising (for a detailed description of these general guidelines, see these books from the Cooper Clinic: *Running Without Fear,*[1] *The Aerobics Program for Total Well-Being,*[2] and *The New Aerobics for Women*[3]). In this chapter I focus on the special problems and hazards people who've had a stroke encounter in exercise.

NINE SAFE-EXERCISE GUIDELINES

The following safety guidelines are intended to reduce the chances that exercise will precipitate another stroke. Following these guidelines will also help prevent exercise-related cardiac complications and musculoskeletal injuries. I encourage you to both follow them and listen to the advice of your doctor.

EXERCISE SAFETY GUIDELINE 1:

Have a thorough medical evaluation before you start your exercise program—and at regular intervals thereafter.

Regardless of age, every stroke patient should have a complete medical exam, including an exercise test, and obtain his or her doctor's permission before beginning this, or any other, exercise program. For a complete rundown of what your pre-exercise screening exam should entail, see Appendix B.

For some stroke patients, the risks of exercise may outweigh the benefits. The contraindications to exercise are outlined in the following checklist.

Do *NOT* Exercise if Your Physician Indicates You Have Any
✓   of These Conditions   ✓

Stroke patients with any of these conditions should avoid aerobic exercise until therapy or the passage of time controls or corrects it. Ask your doctor to let you know if you have any of the following:

_____ A recent TIA or mild stroke that has not been fully investigated or treated

_____ A recent embolism that has not been adequately investigated or treated

_____ Suspected or known aneurysm—cardiac or vascular—that your physician thinks may be worsened by any kind of exertion

_____ Unstable angina pectoris or a recent severe heart attack

_____ Recent significant change in resting ECG that has yet to be fully investigated

_____ Thrombophlebitis or an intracardiac thrombus

_____ Active or suspected myocarditis or pericarditis

_____ Uncontrolled heart failure

_____ Moderate to severe aortic stenosis

_____ Clinically significant hypertrophic obstructive cardiomyopathy

_____ Uncontrolled atrial or ventricular arrhythmias that are considered to be clinically significant

_____ Resting heart rate greater than 120 beats per minute

_____ Third-degree heart block

_____ Uncontrolled hypertension with resting systolic blood pressure above 180 mmHg or diastolic blood pressure above 105 mmHg

_____ Recent fall in systolic blood pressure of more than 20 mmHg that was not caused by medication

_____ Uncontrolled metabolic disease, such as diabetes mellitus, thyrotoxicosis, or myxedema

_____ Acute illness or fever

_____ Chronic infectious disease (such as mononucleosis, hepatitis, or AIDS) that your physician thinks may be worsened by exertion

_____ Significant electrolyte disturbances

_____ Major emotional distress (psychosis)

_____ Neuromuscular, musculoskeletal, or rheumatoid disorders that your physician thinks may be worsened by exertion

_____ Pregnancy complications

_____ Any other condition known to preclude exercise

Note. Adapted from American College of Sports Medicine: Guidelines for Exercise Testing and Prescription, 4th edition. Philadelphia, Lea and Febiger, 1991. Used with permission.

Of course, your pre-exercise medical exam won't be your last. Periodic checkups are important because the conditions that cause a stroke are chronic and often progressive. No one can accurately predict what course your health may take. Nor can anyone guess the exact impact of regular exercise on your body.

The central principle of stroke rehabilitation is that therapies must be continually modified based on the patient's response. Exercise is a form of therapy. That's why I think a reevaluation after 12 weeks on an exercise program is important. It gives your physician the chance to modify your exercise program if necessary. In addition to a physical examination and a talk with your doctor, this follow-up exam should include a reassessment of your range of motion, strength, and aerobic fitness. It should also include a repeat exercise test and any other tests your doctor deems important. (See Appendix B.)

If no disturbing abnormalities are detected, your exercise-related checkups can be annual thereafter. But if you notice disturbing symptoms at any time between regularly scheduled doctor visits, do not hesitate to get an immediate appointment to have them looked into.

EXERCISE SAFETY GUIDELINE 2:

In the beginning, exercise in a program that offers direct medical supervision.

Nearly all stroke survivors can safely do carefully tailored range-of-motion and muscle-strengthening exercises. But there's no getting around the fact that for selected stroke patients, more strenuous aerobic exercise may be too risky. For still other stroke patients, aerobic exercise may be possible—*but only under special medically supervised conditions.*

A *medically supervised* exercise program has three characteristics: A medical doctor helped develop the program. A doctor or other appropriately qualified health professional (such as a physical therapist, exercise physiologist, or nurse) is present and overseeing a patient's actual exercise. And, should the need arise, on-site emergency medical care is instantly available. In contrast, a *medically directed* program is one developed by a doctor but undertaken by a patient at home or a facility where there's no health-care professional standing by. The trend is toward medically directed exercise for reasons that have little to do with medicine. It's generally only large communities that have medically supervised rehabilitation exercise programs, which, when they are available, may be expensive and not scheduled at universally convenient times.

It's trends like this one that make our series of exercise rehabilitation books a necessity. But I encourage you, as a stroke patient, to *begin your exercise under medical supervision, at least for the first 12 weeks. This is crucial if your stroke took place within the last year or if you also have any other serious chronic disease.* Perhaps there is no special program for stroke survivors in your community, but there may be a cardiac rehabilitation program you can join. If 12 weeks in such a program is beyond your budget or impossible for some other reason, get involved for a shorter time. Even one medically supervised session is better than none at all.

In the best of worlds, a stroke patient would continue to exercise with on-site medical supervision indefinitely. In lieu of that, here is some advice:

- Assuming you've completed 12 weeks in a medically supervised program, try to return there for a workout at least once every 3 months, more often if possible. Use the session as an opportunity to review your self-regulated training program with the professional staff members.
- Try to maintain regular telephone or mail contact with the facility. You'll be glad you kept this channel of communication open when you have questions or concerns or you just need motivation to continue exercising.
- Exercise with other people. Group participation, even when it's unsupervised, increases the likelihood you'll stick with your program. It also means that there's someone around who can help you if necessary. Just make sure your companions aren't gung-ho competitive, causing you to go against your better judgment and overdo it.

EXERCISE SAFETY GUIDELINE 3:

Know the warning signs of a stroke. Should you experience any, seek immediate medical care.

Exercise is safe for most stroke patients, *provided it's performed in an appropriate manner.*[4] That's my key point in this book. But there's no denying that once you've had a stroke, you're at an

Steps to take after completing 12 weeks in a medically supervised program

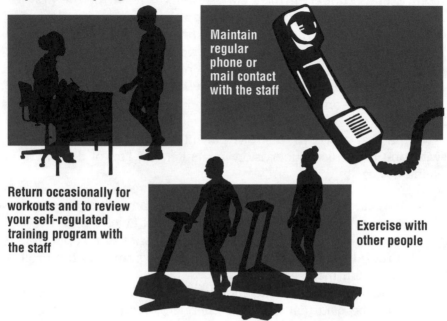

Maintain regular phone or mail contact with the staff

Return occasionally for workouts and to review your self-regulated training program with the staff

Exercise with other people

increased risk for having another one. It happens rarely, but exercise has been known to trigger strokes, particularly hemorrhagic ones, in susceptible people.[5]

About 10% of all strokes are preceded by a TIA. Should you experience a TIA (see chapter 1 for a description of TIAs), take it seriously; about 36% of people who've had one or more TIAs eventually have an ischemic stroke.[6] There's no set pattern to the interval between a TIA and an actual stroke, however. It can be days, weeks, even months. Thus, a TIA is useful for predicting *if* you'll have another stroke, not *when*. The good news is that a TIA does not make an ischemic stroke inevitable—that is, if you treat it as an urgent medical matter demanding immediate evaluation and treatment.

The following box lists the symptoms of a TIA. Unfortunately, these are the same symptoms that accompany a full-fledged ischemic stroke. Should you experience them, don't try to figure out whether you're having a TIA or stroke. Rather, get emergency medical treatment. If you are having another stroke, prompt action may save your life or, at the very least, help limit the brain damage.

WARNING SIGNS OF A TIA EPISODE

A transient ischemic attack happens fast and is usually over quickly. Symptoms become fully expressed within 2 to 5 minutes after you first feel them. Most commonly, an episode will last for more than 2 minutes but less than 15. A spell of only a few seconds duration, though, is probably not a TIA.

- Paralysis, sudden weakness, clumsiness, or loss of sensation in an arm, leg, or the side of your face. You may experience a single symptom in one place or most of these symptoms in several places.
- Loss of vision.
- Loss of speech or difficulty in speaking or in understanding what others are saying.
- Loss of balance, dizziness, unsteadiness, double vision, or difficulty in swallowing. When these symptoms are the only ones, you may not be experiencing a TIA.

Source: Adapted from the American Heart Association booklet *1990 Heart and Stroke Facts*; and National Institute of Neurological Disorders and Stroke, "Classification of Cerebrovascular Disease III." *Stroke*, 21 (1990): 637-676.

In contrast to ischemic strokes, hemorrhagic strokes give little warning and are seldom preceded by a TIA. By the time you feel the symptoms (frequently a sudden, severe headache and a sensation of fainting), you're having the stroke. You may also vomit and lose consciousness for a few minutes. Urgent medical care is needed.[7]

EXERCISE SAFETY GUIDELINE 4:

Be thoroughly versed in the warning signs of an impending cardiac complication.

You're probably far more likely to die from the deleterious effects of sedentary living than you are to die from a heart attack during exercise. But I know stroke patients worry a lot about this, and I agree it's prudent to keep your cardiac risk as low as reasonably possible. One of the best ways to boost your exercise benefit-to-risk ratio is to remember this axiom:

Although death from a heart attack during exercise is always unexpected, it's seldom unheralded.

In other words, often you'll have some warning if things are awry with your heart. The following box lists these signs. Pay special heed because people with heart disease are at the greatest risk for exercise-induced cardiac problems, and about 65% of people who have had a stroke have some form of heart disease.[8] If you experience any of these symptoms before, during, or just after exercise, discuss them with your doctor before continuing with exercise.

WARNING SIGNS OF HEART PROBLEMS

✓ *Pain or discomfort in your chest, abdomen, back, neck, jaw, or arms.* Such symptoms may be signs of an inadequate supply of blood and oxygen to your heart muscle because of potentially serious conditions such as atherosclerotic plaque buildup in your coronary arteries.

✓ *A nauseous sensation during or after exercise.* This can result from a variety of causes, but it can also signify a cardiac abnormality.

✓ *Unaccustomed shortness of breath during exercise.* Any kind of aerobic exercise may make you huff and puff. This isn't what I'm referring to here. Let's say an ordinary part of your routine is to walk 2 miles (3.2 kilometers) in 45 minutes with no breathlessness. If one day you can't do it anymore, you should be alarmed.

✓ *Dizziness or fainting.* This can occur in perfectly healthy people who don't follow proper exercise protocol and fail to cool down adequately. Anyone could feel dizzy momentarily or even actually faint if he or she stops exercising suddenly. The type of dizziness I'm concerned about occurs while you're exercising rather than upon stopping suddenly. This is a more probable sign of a serious heart problem and warrants immediate medical consultation.

✓ *An irregular pulse, particularly when it's been regular in your past exercise sessions.* If you notice what appears to be extra heartbeats or skipped beats, notify your doctor. This too might not be anything of significance; on the other hand, it could point to heart problems.

✓ *A very rapid heart rate at rest.* This means 100 beats per minute or higher after at least 5 minutes of rest. Although this could result from a variety of causes, including a fever, it can also point to cardiac abnormalities. It should be reported to your doctor.

EXERCISE SAFETY GUIDELINE 5:

Put safety at the top of your exercise priority list by following proper exercise protocol.

When it comes to exercise, there's a right way and a wrong way to do it, a safe way and a dangerous way. As I've mentioned, even healthy people should follow safety guidelines when exercising. The following guidelines have special relevance for exercisers who have had a stroke:

• *Warm up and cool down adequately—a minimum of 5 minutes for each.* Sufficient warm-up and cool-down are important for every exerciser but especially for stroke patients. More than 70% of cardiac problems that surface during exercise do so either at the beginning or at the end of a session.[9]

• *Don't exercise in adverse climatic conditions, particularly without taking adequate precautions.* In warm weather, you'll want to avoid hyperthermia, an overheating of the body during exercise. It not only impairs your ability to exercise but also predisposes you to heatstroke, a potentially fatal condition. The symptoms of hyperthermia include headache, dizziness, confusion, stumbling, nausea, cramps, cessation of sweating, or excessive sweating. To avoid hyperthermia, here are four preventive measures you can take:

- Let both heat and humidity guide your decision about when outdoor exercise is appropriate. Don't engage in strenuous exercise when they're both high.
- Wear clothing that promotes heat loss. Fabrics that "breathe," such as a mesh or fishnet T-shirt, are good choices.
- Drink fluids while you're exercising, especially on hot days. Do this even if you're not thirsty. About 15 minutes before you begin, drink 8 ounces (240 ml) of cold water, which is absorbed more quickly than lukewarm water. If your workout lasts longer than 30 minutes, take another 8-ounce drink at 15- to 20-minute intervals during exercise.
- If you must exercise in the heat, sponge off the exposed parts of your body with cool water at regular intervals.

Symptoms of hyperthermia

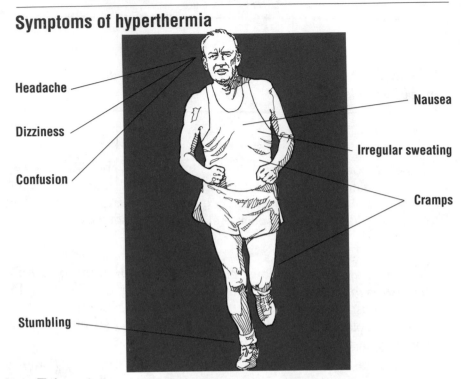

Headache

Dizziness

Confusion

Stumbling

Nausea

Irregular sweating

Cramps

• *Take adequate precautions for cold-weather workouts.* About one third of heart patients report a worsening of their angina symptoms during winter-weather workouts. Choose clothing that provides adequate insulation from the cold, but avoid fabrics that cause excessive buildup of sweat. Multiple layers of clothing are a good choice for cold weather.

Once again, use good judgment about exercising in the cold. Stay indoors when the windchill index falls below 15 °F (−10 °C). If it's icy or slippery, forget about outdoor exercise until more hospitable conditions prevail.[10]

• *Skip exercise when you have a fever, influenza, or other moderately serious acute illness.* (You may not think it's necessary to include this warning. After all, who would want to exercise when sick? Believe it or not, lots of enthusiasts I know do.)

An infectious fever and aerobics are a dubious combination. Exerting yourself heavily while you're fighting an infection (including influenza) can trigger hyperthermia, worsen the infection, and sometimes place you at risk for viral myocarditis, a potentially lethal inflammatory condition of the heart muscle.[11]

If you've got nothing more serious than a cold, go ahead with aerobics if your temperature is normal, your symptoms are above your neck (for example, runny nose, sneezing, scratchy throat), and you feel like it. But when your ailment is more serious, and especially if it's accompanied by fever, sit out aerobics and all other forms of strenuous exercise until you're better. After an illness, ease your way back into aerobics gradually over the course of at least a week or two.

• *Wear quality shoes designed for the specific type of weight-bearing exercise you're doing.* Wearing the right shoes is crucial for anyone who wants to sidestep foot and knee problems and injuries. Technological advances have provided us with a wide selection in exercise shoes. You can buy shoes that are specially designed for a particular sport as well as engineered to suit a specific foot type. You can also help prevent foot and knee problems by performing any high-impact, weight-bearing activities (such as jogging) on a soft rather than a hard, nonresistant surface. For example, choose grass over cement.

EXERCISE SAFETY GUIDELINE 6:

Avoid physical activities that will cause an excessive rise in your blood pressure.

It would seem logical that for people with hypertension (including stroke patients), strenuous exertion would push their blood pressure up to dangerously high levels. It would also seem to follow that such exercisers are at great risk for exercise-induced hemorrhagic strokes. But what seems logical isn't necessarily so. There's no medical proof that these assumptions are accurate.[12, 13]

Still, I think it's prudent for you to avoid a steep rise in your blood pressure during exercise, especially if you've had a hemorrhagic stroke. I consider a systolic blood pressure greater than 220 mmHg or a diastolic blood pressure greater than 110 mmHg during exercise to be too high. Here are types of exercise—or ways of doing an exercise—that can cause a steep rise in blood pressure. To stay on the safe side, you should not undertake the following:

• High-intensity exercise that pushes your heart rate above 85% of your maximal value.
• Anaerobic exercise, such as sprinting, that involves short, intense bursts of exertion.

- Heavy lifting or strength training. Err in the direction of less weight or resistance and more repetitions, not the other way around.
- Muscle contractions that you hold longer than 6 seconds.
- A *Valsalva maneuver*, which involves holding your breath while performing muscle-strengthening exercises.
- Competitive exercise, unless you have special clearance from your doctor.
- Exercises requiring positions where your head is low—for example, a stretching exercise where you lower your head toward the floor. Such movements increase the pressure inside the blood vessels of your brain.

In general, activities that use large muscle groups (for example, walking and stationary cycling) cause less rise in blood pressure than those confined to a few muscles (arm-cycle ergometry, for example). Keep this in mind as you choose your aerobic exercises.

EXERCISE SAFETY GUIDELINE 7:

Don't overestimate your capabilities and undertake potentially risky exercises—especially without adequate assistance.

What do I mean here? Let's say you normally walk with a cane. Don't suddenly try exercising without one. Before you make any radical changes, check with your health-care team and make sure someone is available to assist you the first few times you try it. You don't want to fall and injure yourself.

Falls are especially hazardous for stroke survivors and tricky for them to get up from. Ask your health-care team about falls, in particular how to get up from the floor. I advise stroke patients to rely mainly on their unaffected limbs in doing so, and I have them practice doing it.

EXERCISE SAFETY GUIDELINE 8:

Know the specific precautions to take if you have other chronic diseases. And be aware of how medications alter your body's response to exercise.

If you're elderly and have had a stroke, it's very likely you have other chronic ailments such as heart disease, diabetes, peripheral vascular disease, or arthritis. If you do, it's important that you ask your doctor about any special precautions that you should take. You can also consult other books in this series that deal with your condition.

Prescription medications can be problematic for exercisers— another reason why you should see your doctor before you begin your program. Many stroke patients are on drugs such as beta blockers that alter the heart rate or blood pressure, or both. Make sure you're taking your usual dosage of your medications when you have your exercise test so that it will accurately reflect how your body reacts to exertion. View the test as a simulated exercise session. For example, if you intend to exercise in the late afternoon, 10 hours after taking your medication, then schedule your exercise test in the late afternoon too, or at least at the same interval (10 hours after consuming medication). The point is to mimic the biological conditions you'll experience during a regular exercise workout.[14]

EXERCISE SAFETY GUIDELINE 9:

Monitor improvements or backsliding in your ability to take care of yourself. Contact your doctor promptly should you notice a downtrend.

During the first months after your stroke, your health-care team probably made regular assessments of your functional capacity, your ability to take care of yourself without depending on others. They used these assessments to make decisions about your therapy and to uncover any complications. But once the formal part of your rehabilitation ceased, so probably did these periodic assessments.

I ask our stroke patients who still have disabilities, even mild ones, to keep making such assessments monthly so they'll know how they're progressing. The following chart provides the means to conduct such a self-assessment. It is based on the Barthel Index, which is well known and respected in stroke rehabilitation circles.[15, 16]

(Make photocopies and fill in monthly.)

The Barthel Index:

How Much Is My Stroke Continuing to Interfere With My Ability to Lead a Normal, Independent Life?

By taking this functional capacity test once a month and comparing the results over time, you'll be able to see whether you're making progress or regressing in your quest to return to full self-reliance.

I have control over defecation (my bowels).	0 = never 1 = sometimes 2 = always _____
I have control over urination (my bladder).	0 = never/catheterized and unable to manage 1 = sometimes 2 = always _____
When it comes to grooming myself (face, hair, teeth, shaving), I need help.	0 = always 1 = never _____
To use the toilet, I'm . . .	0 = dependent on others 1 = in need of some help 2 = independent _____
When it comes to feeding myself, I'm . . .	0 = dependent on others 1 = in need of some help (with cutting, spreading butter, etc.) 2 = independent _____

To get into and out of chairs and bed, I'm . . .	0 = unable to sit and dependent on others for transfers 1 = able to sit but need a lot of help for transfers 2 = need a little help for transfers 3 = independent _____
Concerning walking, I . . .	0 = cannot; I'm confined to a wheelchair that others operate 1 = cannot; although I'm in a wheelchair, I can operate it myself 2 = can but only with the physical or verbal assistance of others 3 = am fully independent and need no help from other people _____
To dress, I'm . . .	0 = dependent on others 1 = in need of some help 2 = independent; I can deal with buttons, zippers, shoe laces, etc. _____
When it comes to climbing stairs, I'm . . .	0 = unable 1 = in need of help 2 = independent _____
To bathe, I'm . . .	0 = dependent on others 1 = independent; I need no help, including getting into and out of the bathtub _____
	Total _____

Monthly Score

Once a month, transfer the scores above to the corresponding boxes below.

Functional categories	Jan.	Feb.	March	April	May	June	July	Aug.	Sept.	Oct.	Nov.	Dec.
Defecation												
Urination												
Grooming												
Toilet use												
Feeding												
Chair/bed transfers												
Walking												
Dressing												
Stairs												
Bathing												
Total each month												

Score Interpretation

Over the course of several months, you'll be able to evaluate whether your functional capacity is improving or going downhill. If your scores are getting consistently worse, I suggest you talk to your doctor about altering your treatment and rehabilitation program.

Monthly point totals representing functional capacity	*Interpretation*
0-4	Very severely disabled
5-9	Severely disabled
10-14	Moderately disabled
15-19	Mildly disabled
20	Independent and fully functional

Adapted from: D.T. Wade, R. Langton Hewer, "Functional Abilities After Stroke: Measurement, Natural History and Prognosis." *Journal of Neurology, Neurosurgery, and Psychiatry*, 50 (1987): 177-182.

SOME CONCLUDING THOUGHTS

In this book, I've offered you a state-of-the-art method for using regular exercise to reduce your disability and optimize both the quality and the quantity of your life. My advice is based on what is currently known about exercise and strokes. In years to come, far more will be learned about how stroke patients, such as you, can benefit the most from an exercise rehabilitation program. But don't wait until then to begin a physically active lifestyle. Now is the time for you, in consultation with your doctor, to plan your program from the prototype I've provided.

The sooner you begin a sensible exercise program, the sooner you will reap the many rewards. Once you get started, never forget that exercise should be fun. I've always enjoyed it thoroughly and have no doubt that with time you will too.

Good luck! And the best of health to you.

Chapter 5

Prescription

- ❐ Have a thorough medical evaluation before you start your exercise program—and at regular intervals thereafter.
- ❐ In the beginning, exercise in a program that offers direct medical supervision if possible.
- ❐ Know the warning signs of a stroke. Should you experience any, seek immediate medical care.
- ❐ Know the warning signs of an impending cardiac complication.
- ❐ Don't exercise in adverse climatic conditions, particularly without taking adequate precautions.
- ❐ Skip exercise when you have a fever, influenza, or other moderately serious acute illness.
- ❐ Wear quality shoes designed for the specific type of weight-bearing exercise you are doing.
- ❐ Avoid physical activities that will cause an excessive rise in your blood pressure.
- ❐ Don't overestimate your capabilities and undertake potentially risky exercises—especially without adequate assistance.
- ❐ Know the specific precautions to take if you have any other chronic disease. And be aware of how medications alter your body's response to exercise.
- ❐ Monitor improvements or backsliding in your ability to take care of yourself. Contact your doctor promptly should you notice a downtrend.

Appendix A

How to Take Your Pulse and Calculate Your Heart Rate

You have two pulse points to choose from—the radial artery in your wrist or the carotid artery in your throat. Your radial artery is the preferred place because the reading there is usually more accurate.

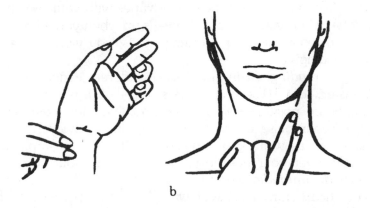

a   b

Figure A.1 Pulse points: a) radial artery, b) carotid artery. *Note.* From *ACSM Fitness Book* (p. 24) by The American College of Sports Medicine, 1992, Champaign, IL: Leisure Press. Copyright 1992 by The American College of Sports Medicine. Reprinted by permission.

Your two carotid arteries are located on either side of your windpipe. These arteries are large, and you should be able to locate them easily by gently pressing just to the right or left of your Adam's apple. But there are several things you must keep in mind. Don't press hard; press on only one carotid artery at a time; and do not press too near the jawbone. If you do any of these things your heart rate may slow down excessively and result in potentially harmful consequences, not to mention an inaccurate reading.

Taking your pulse is a three-step process. Here are instructions for taking a wrist pulse reading. Resort to your carotid artery only if you absolutely cannot locate the radial artery in your wrist.

1. *Locate the pulse in your wrist.* The hand of your wristwatch arm is the one you will use to monitor the pulse in your opposite wrist. Your "sensors" are the pads of your fingers, not your fingertips.

Place your index finger and middle finger at the base of the outer third of your wrist, the side on which your thumb is located. If you feel your wrist's tendons, you need to move your fingers further to the outside of your wrist. Do this incrementally, changing the location of your fingers by about a quarter of an inch until you finally locate a pulsation. Don't press too hard or you may obliterate your pulse. A light but firm pressure is all that is needed. You should be able to feel your pulse each time your heart beats, thus making your pulse rate equivalent to your heart rate.

2. *Count your pulse.* To determine your *resting heart rate*, count for 30 to 60 seconds. Your heart rate varies with your breathing; it slows down when you exhale and speeds up when you inhale. Thus, if you count your pulse for shorter periods, you won't get a good average reading.

Taking a reading during exercise is different. Then your pulse rate is faster, so a 10-second count is sufficient. If you're exercising in a stationary position—on a cycle ergometer, for example—you can count your pulse easily without stopping. However, if you're moving—such as walking or jogging—you'll need to stop, but not completely. Keep your legs moving while you take your pulse, which *you must do immediately*. If you wait for more than a second or two, your heart starts to slow down. This is true particularly if you are fit. If you count for longer than 10 seconds, you run the risk of greatly *underestimating* your heart rate.

When counting your pulse, count as "one" the first pulsation you feel *after* your watchhand hits a digit. Do *not* count as "one" any pulsation that occurs at the same time as the hand hits the digit. Continue the count until your watch registers 10 seconds. If a pulsation occurs at the same time as the watchhand hits the 10-second point, count it, but none thereafter.

3. *Calculate your heart rate.* After you've counted your pulse for 10 seconds, multiply that number by 6 to get your heart rate (beats per minute). Here's a chart with the calculations already done for 10-second pulse counts of 12 through 31:

12 = 72	17 = 102	22 = 132	27 = 162
13 = 78	18 = 108	23 = 138	28 = 168
14 = 84	19 = 114	24 = 144	29 = 174
15 = 90	20 = 120	25 = 150	30 = 180
16 = 96	21 = 126	26 = 156	31 = 186

Tests and Procedures Included in a Thorough Pre-Exercise Medical Exam for Stroke Survivors

H ere I describe what happens during a typical medical exam for a stroke survivor. Use this checklist to assure yourself that your physician has been thorough.

✓   **Checkup Checklist**   ✓

_____ My physician or physician's assistant takes a thorough medical history to identify diseases or symptoms suggestive of disease. They probe my attitudes about exercise and stroke in general, as well as my ability to perform the physical activities of daily living. Finally, they document all the medications I'm taking that could possibly interact with exercise in any way.

I'm examined for various illnesses. In particular, I'm given a thorough cardiovascular and neurologic exam, which includes these items:

_____ Measuring my blood pressure in both arms and while I'm lying, sitting, and standing.

_____ Monitoring the pulses in my neck, arms, and legs.

_____ Listening to my neck, chest, heart, abdomen, and femoral arteries in my groin with a stethoscope.

_____ Testing my reflexes, muscle tone, and sensation.

_____ Examining my eyes (the doctor looks inside my eyes with a special light, or *ophthalmoscope*).

_____ Taking a chest X ray, if I haven't had one recently.

_____ Taking a blood-lipid profile (which goes much farther than a mere total cholesterol count), if I haven't had one recently.

_____ Taking a fasting blood-glucose measurement, if I haven't had one recently.

_____ Taking a resting electrocardiogram (ECG).

_____ Administering an exercise test (known as a *symptom-limited maximal exercise test*) with ECG and blood-pressure monitoring. The purpose is to assess my cardiovascular response to exercise in order to tailor an exercise program that's safe and effective for me and to measure my current level of aerobic fitness. Ideally, this test is performed with me walking on a treadmill or riding a stationary cycle, using my legs alone or both legs and arms. If I'm not capable of these options, the test is performed using arm-cycle ergometry. If necessary, the exercise testing equipment is specially adapted to accommodate my disabilities.

_____ I'm checked for any musculoskeletal problems that may limit my ability to exercise or that exercise could make worse.

_____ My body weight and, if possible, percentage body fat are measured.

_____ My joints are given range-of-motion and flexibility assessments of both the active and passive kind. An active evaluation means I move my joint through its full range of motion. A passive assessment means that I remain relaxed and my doctor or physical therapist provides the locomotion to move my joint.

_____ My physician checks my body's muscular strength, with or without sophisticated equipment. (Strength tests done with equipment such as a Cybex isokinetic dynamometer generally provide more objective and complete information.)

_____ My physician reviews the results of all pertinent previous tests I've had (for example, CAT scans, MRIs, angiograms, heart catheterizations, or echocardiograms).

_____ My physician performs any other additional tests that he or she feels are necessary, given my specific circumstances.

Notes

FOREWORD

[1]Black-Schaffer, R.M., and Osberg, G.S. "Return to Work After Stroke: Development of a Predictive Model." *Archives of Physical Medicine and Rehabilitation* 71 (1990): 285-290.

[2]American Heart Association. Fact Sheet on Heart Attack, Stroke and Risk Factors. Dallas: American Heart Association, 1991.

[3]Bonita, R., Stewart, A., and Beaglehole, R. "International Trends in Stroke Mortality: 1970-1985." *Stroke* 21 (1990): 989-992.

CHAPTER 1

[1]Moser, M. *Lower Your Blood Pressure and Live Longer.* New York: Villard Books, 1989: xv-xvi.

[2]Cooper, K., and Cooper, M. *The New Aerobics for Women.* New York: Bantam Books, 1988: 284-286.

[3]World Health Organization. "Stroke—1989: Recommendations on Stroke Prevention, Diagnosis, and Therapy." *Stroke* 20 (1989): 1407-1431.

[4]Nadeau, S.E. "Stroke." *Medical Clinics of North America* 73 (1989): 1351-1369.

[5]National Stroke Association. *Stroke: Putting the Pieces Back Together.* Englewood, CO: National Stroke Association, 1990.

[6]Brandstater, M.E. "An Overview of Stroke Rehabilitation." *Stroke* 21 (1990): II-40-II-41.

[7]Dombovy, M.L., et al. "Disability and Use of Rehabilitation Services Following Stroke in Rochester, Minnesota, 1975-1979." *Stroke* 18 (1987): 830-836.

CHAPTER 2

[1]Wade, D.T., et al. *Stroke: A Critical Approach to Diagnosis, Treatment, and Management.* Chicago: Year Book Medical Publishers, Inc., 1985.

[2]World Health Organization. "Stroke—1989: Recommendations on Stroke Prevention, Diagnosis, and Therapy." *Stroke* 20 (1989): 1407-1431.

[3]Tangeman, P.T., Banaitis, D.A., and Williams, A.K. "Rehabilitation of Chronic Stroke Patients: Changes in Functional Performance." *Archives of Physical Medicine and Rehabilitation* 71 (1990): 876-880.

[4]Ades, P.A., and Grunvald, M.H. "Cardiopulmonary Exercise Testing Before and After Conditioning in Older Coronary Patients." *American Heart Journal* 120 (1990): 585-589.

[5]Jankowski, L.W., and Sullivan, S.J. "Aerobic and Neuromuscular Training: Effect on the Capacity, Efficiency and Fatigability of Patients With Traumatic Brain Injuries." *Archives of Physical Medicine and Rehabilitation* 71 (1990): 500-504.

[6]Bouchard, C., et al., eds. *Exercise, Fitness, and Health.* Champaign, IL: Human Kinetics, 1990.

[7]American Heart Association. *1990 Heart and Stroke Facts.* Dallas: American Heart Association, 1990.

[8]Goldberg, G., and Berger, G.G. "Secondary Prevention in Stroke: A Primary Rehabilitation Concern." *Archives of Physical Medicine and Rehabilitation* 69 (1988): 32-40.

[9]Paffenbarger, Jr., R.S., and Wing, A.L. "Characteristics in Youth Predisposing to Fatal Stroke in Later Years." *Lancet* 1 (1967): 753-754.

[10]Hammond, E.C., and Garfinkel, L. "Coronary Heart Disease, Stroke, and Aortic Aneurysm: Factors in the Etiology." *Archives of Environmental Health* 19 (1969): 167-182.

[11]Salonen, J.T., Puska, P., and Tuomilehto, J. "Physical Activity and Risk of Myocardial Infarction, Cerebral Stroke and Death." *American Journal of Epidemiology* 115 (1982): 526-537.

[12]Lapidus, L., and Bengtsson, C. "Socioeconomic Factors and Physical Activity in Relation to Cardiovascular Disease and Death." *British Heart Journal* 55 (1986): 295-301.

[13]Paffenbarger, Jr., R.S., et al. "A Natural History of Athleticism and Cardiovascular Health." *Journal of the American Medical Association* 252 (1986): 491-495.

[14]Blair, S.N., Kohl, H.W., and Barlow, C.E. "Low Cardiorespiratory Fitness and Incidence of Non-Fatal Stroke." *Medicine and Science in Sports and Exercise* 21 (1989): 849.

[15]Work, G. "Low Fitness May Mean Higher Risk of Stroke." *Physician and Sportsmedicine* 17 (1989): 37-40.

[16]Roth, E.J., Mueller, K., and Green, D. "Stroke Rehabilitation Outcome: Impact of Coronary Artery Disease." *Stroke* 19 (1988): 42-47.

[17]Berlin, G.A., and Colditz, G.A. "A Meta-Analysis of Physical Activity in the Prevention of Coronary Artery Disease." *American Journal of Epidemiology* 132 (1990): 612-628.

[18]Oldridge, N.B., et al. "Cardiac Rehabilitation After Myocardial Infarction." *Journal of the American Medical Association* 260 (1988): 945-950.

[19]U.S. Preventive Services Task Force. *Guide to Clinical Preventive Services*. Baltimore: Williams & Wilkins, 1989.

[20]Gordon, N.F., et al. "Exercise and Mild Essential Hypertension: Recommendations for Adults." *Sports Medicine* 10 (1990): 390-404.

[21]Gordon, N.F., and Scott, C.B. "Exercise and Mild Hypertension." *Primary Care* 18 (1991): 683-694.

[22]Niemi, M.L., et al. "Quality of Life 4 Years After Stroke." *Stroke* 19 (1988): 1101-1107.

[23]Santus, G., et al. "Social and Family Integration of Hemiplegic Elderly Patients 1 Year After Stroke." *Stroke* 21 (1990): 1019-1022.

[24]Raglin, G.S. "Exercise and Mental Health: Beneficial and Detrimental Effects." *Sports Medicine* 9 (1990): 323-329.

[25]Sidney, K.H., and Jerome, W.C. "Anxiety and Depression: Exercise for Mood Enhancement." In *Current Therapy in Sports Medicine—2*, edited by J.S. Torg et al. Toronto: B.C. Decker, Inc., 1990.

[26]Parikh, R.M., et al. "The Impact of Poststroke Depression on Recovery in Activities of Daily Living Over a 2-Year Follow-Up." *Archives of Neurology* 47 (1990): 785-789.

[27]Rusin, M.J. "Stroke Rehabilitation: A Geropsychological Perspective." *Archives of Physical Medicine and Rehabilitation* 71 (1990): 914-922.

[28]Gibbons, L.W., et al. "The Safety of Maximal Exercise Testing." *Circulation* 80 (1989): 846-852.

[29]Gibbons, L.W., et al. "The Acute Cardiac Risk of Strenuous Exercise." *Journal of the American Medical Association* 244 (1980): 1799-1801.

[30]Thompson, P.D., et al. "Incidence of Death During Jogging in Rhode Island from 1975 Through 1980." *Journal of the American Medical Association* 274 (1982): 2535-2538.

[31]Chester, J.F., and Conlon, C.P. "Some Cerebrovascular Complications of Exercise." *British Journal of Sports Medicine* 17 (1983): 143-144.

[32]Van Camp, S.P., and Peterson, R.A. "Cardiovascular Complications of Outpatient Cardiac Rehabilitation Programs." *Journal of the American Medical Association* 256 (1986): 1160-1163.

[33]Macera, C., et al. "Predicting Lower-Extremity Injuries Among Habitual Runners." *Archives of Internal Medicine* 149 (1989): 2565-2568.

[34]Walter, S., et al. "The Ontario Cohort Study of Running-Related Injuries." *Archives of Internal Medicine* 149 (1989): 2561-2564.

[35]Blair, S.N., Kohl, H.W., and Goodyear, N.N. "Rates and Risks for Running and Exercise Injuries: Studies in Three Populations." *Research Quarterly for Exercise and Sport* 58 (1987): 221-228.

CHAPTER 3

[1]Institute for Aerobics Research. *The Strength Connection*. Dallas: Institute for Aerobics Research, 1990.

[2]Wolf, S.L., et al. "Forced Use of Hemiplegic Upper Extremities to Reverse the Effect of Learned Nonuse Among Chronic Stroke and Head-Injured Patients." *Experimental Neurology* 104 (1989): 125-132.

[3]Sherman, D.G., Hart, R.G., and Easton, J.D. "Abrupt Change in Head Position and Cerebral Infarction." *Stroke* 12 (1981): 2-6.

[4]Pryse-Phillips, W. "Infarction of the Medulla and Cervical Cord After Fitness Exercises." *Stroke* 20 (1989): 292-294.

[5]MacDougall, J.D., et al. "Arterial Blood Pressure Response to Heavy Resistance Exercise." *Journal of Applied Physiology* 58 (1985): 785-790.

[6]Tipton, C.M., et al. "Response of Hypertensive Rats to Acute and Chronic Conditions of Static Exercise." *American Journal of Physiology* 254 (1988): H592-H598.

[7]Gordon, N.F., et al. "Exercise and Mild Essential Hypertension: Recommendations for Adults." *Sports Medicine* 10 (1990): 390-404.

[8]American Association of Cardiovascular and Pulmonary Rehabilitation. *Guidelines for Cardiac Rehabilitation Programs*. Champaign, IL: Human Kinetics, 1991.

[9]Inaba, M., et al. "Effectiveness of Functional Training, Active Exercise, and Resistive Exercise for Patients With Hemiplegia." *Physical Therapy* 53 (1973): 28-35.

[10]Agre, J.C., et al. "Light Resistance and Stretching Exercise in Elderly Women: Effect Upon Strength." *Archives of Physical Medicine and Rehabilitation* 69 (1988): 273-276.

[11]American College of Sports Medicine. "Position Stand: The Recommended Quantity and Quality of Exercise for Developing and Maintaining Cardiorespiratory and Muscular Fitness in Healthy Adults." *Medicine and Science in Sports and Exercise* 22 (1990): 265-274.

[12]American College of Sports Medicine. *Guidelines for Exercise Testing and Prescription*. Philadelphia: Lea & Febiger, 1991.

[13]Cooper, K.H. *Aerobics*. New York: Bantam Books, 1968.

[14]Blair, S.N., et al. "Exercise and Fitness in Childhood: Implications for a Lifetime of Health." In *Perspective in Exercise Science and Sports Medicine—2: Youth, Exercise and Sport*, edited by C.V. Gisolfi and D.R. Lamb. Indianapolis: Benchmark Press, 1989: 401-430.

[15]American Heart Association. "Exercise Standards: A Statement for Health Professionals from the American Heart Association." *Circulation* 82 (1990): 2286-2322.

[16]Haskell, W.L., Montoye, H.J., and Orenstein, D. "Physical Activity and Exercise to Achieve Health-Related Physical Fitness Components." *Public Health Reports* 100 (1985): 202-212.

[17]Blair, S.N. *Living With Exercise*. Dallas: American Health Publishing Co., 1991.

[18]DeBusk, R.F., et al. "Training Effects of Long Versus Short Bouts of Exercise in Healthy Subjects." *American Journal of Cardiology* 65 (1990) : 1010-1013.

[19]Borg, G.A. "Psychophysical Bases of Perceived Exertion." *Medicine and Science in Sports and Exercise* 14 (1982): 377-387.

[20]Katz, S., et al. "Progress After Strokes: Part II. Long-Term Course of 159 Patients." *Medicine* 45 (1966): 236-246.

[21]Thomas, T.R., and Londeree, B.R. "Energy Cost During Prolonged Walking Vs. Jogging Exercise." *Physician and Sportsmedicine* 17 (1989): 93-102.

[22]National Stroke Association. *The Road Ahead: A Stroke Recovery Guide.* Englewood, CO: National Stroke Association, 1989.

[23]Yanker, G., and Burton, K. *Walking Medicine.* New York: McGraw-Hill, 1990.

[24]King, M.L., et al. "Adaptive Exercise Testing for Patients With Hemiparesis." *Journal of Cardiopulmonary Rehabilitation* 9 (1989): 237-242.

[25]Curtis, K.A., and Dillon, D.A. "Survey of Wheelchair Athletic Injuries: Common Patterns and Prevention." *Paraplegia* 23 (1985): 170-175.

[26]Glaser, R.M., and Davis, G.M. "Wheelchair-Dependent Individuals." In *Exercise in Modern Medicine,* edited by B.A. Franklin, S. Gordon, and G.C. Timmis. Baltimore: Williams & Wilkins, 1989: 237-267.

CHAPTER 4

[1]Bard, G. "Energy Expenditure of Hemiplegic Subjects During Walking." *Archives of Physical Medicine and Rehabilitation* 44 (1963): 368-370.

[2]Fisher, S.V., and Gullickson, G. "Energy Cost of Ambulation in Health and Disability: A Literature Review." *Archives of Physical Medicine and Rehabilitation* 59 (1978): 124-133.

[3]Koszuta, L.E. "Water Exercise Causes Ripples." *Physician and Sportsmedicine* 14 (1986): 163-167.

[4]Cooper, K.H. *Overcoming Hypertension.* New York: Bantam Books, 1990.

[5]Cooper, K.H. *The Aerobics Program for Total Well-Being.* New York: Bantam Books, 1982.

[6]DeBenedette, V. "Stair Machines: The Truth About This Fitness Fad." *Physician and Sportsmedicine* 18 (1990): 131-134.

[7]Gordon, N.F., Kohl, H.W., and Villegas, J.A. "Effects of Rest Interval Duration on Cardiorespiratory Responses to Hydraulic Resistance Circuit Training." *Journal of Cardiopulmonary Rehabilitation* 9 (1989): 325-330.

[8]Paffenbarger, Jr., R.S., et al. "Physical Activity, All-Cause Mortality, and Longevity in College Alumni." *New England Journal of Medicine* 314 (1986): 605-613.

[9]Coyle, E.F. "Detraining and Retension of Training-Induced Adaptations." In *Resource Manual for Guidelines for Exercise Testing and Prescription,* edited by S.N. Blair, et al. Philadelphia: Lea & Febiger, 1988.

CHAPTER 5

[1]Cooper, K.H. *Running Without Fear*. New York: M. Evans & Co., 1985.

[2]Cooper, K.H. *The Aerobics Program for Total Well-Being*. New York: Bantam Books, 1982.

[3]Cooper, K.H., and Cooper, M. *The New Aerobics for Women*. New York: Bantam Books, 1988.

[4]Monga, T.N., et al. "Cardiovascular Responses to Acute Exercise in Patients With Cerebrovascular Accidents." *Archives of Physical Medicine and Rehabilitation* 69 (1988): 937-940.

[5]Lynch, P. "Soldiers, Sport, and Sudden Death." *Lancet* 1 (1980): 1235-1237.

[6]American Heart Association. *1990 Heart and Stroke Facts*. Dallas: American Heart Association, 1990.

[7]National Institute of Neurological Disorders and Stroke. "Classification of Cerebrovascular Disease III." *Stroke* 21 (1990): 637-676.

[8]National Stroke Association. *Stroke: Putting the Pieces Back Together*. Englewood, CO: National Stroke Association, 1990.

[9]Monga, T.N., et al. "Cardiovascular Responses to Acute Exercise in Patients With Cerebrovascular Accidents." *Archives of Physical Medicine and Rehabilitation* 69 (1988): 937-940.

[10]Gordon, N.F., and Gibbons, L.W. *The Cooper Clinic Cardiac Rehabilitation Program*. New York: Simon & Schuster, 1990.

[11]Ilback, N.G., Fohlman, J., and Friman, G. "Exercise in Coxsackie B3 Myocarditis: Effects on Heart Lymphocyte Subpopulations and the Inflammatory Reaction." *American Heart Journal* 117 (1989): 1298-1302.

[12]Frohlich, E.D., et al. "Task Force IV: Systemic Arterial Hypertension." *Journal of the American College of Cardiology* 6 (1985): 1218-1221.

[13]Pickering, T.G. "Pathology of Exercise Hypertension." *Herz* 12 (1987): 119-124.

[14]American College of Sports Medicine. *Guidelines for Exercise Testing and Prescription*. Philadelphia: Lea & Febiger, 1991.

[15]Wade, D.T., and Langton Hewer, R. "Functional Abilities After Stroke: Measurement, Natural History and Prognosis." *Journal of Neurology, Neurosurgery, and Psychiatry* 50 (1987): 177-182.

[16]Gresham, G.E., Phillips, T.F., and Labi, M.L.C. "ADL Status in Stroke: Relative Merits of Three Standard Indexes." *Archives of Physical Medicine and Rehabilitation* 61 (1980): 355-358.

Index